VITAMIN C

Everything
You Need
to Know

Other Books From the People's Medical Society

VITAMIN C

Everything
You Need
to Know

By Jennifer Hay

≡People's Medical Society®

Allentown, Pennsylvania

The People's Medical Society is a nonprofit consumer health organization dedicated to the principles of better, more responsive and less expensive medical care. Organized in 1983, the People's Medical Society puts previously unavailable medical information into the hands of consumers so that they can make informed decisions about their own health care.

Membership in the People's Medical Society is $20 a year and includes a subscription to the *People's Medical Society Newsletter.* For information, write to the People's Medical Society, 462 Walnut Street, Allentown, PA 18102, or call 610-770-1670.

This and other People's Medical Society publications are available for quantity purchase at discount. Contact the People's Medical Society for details.

Many of the designations used by manufacturers and sellers to distinguish their products are claimed as trademarks. Where those designations appear in this book and the People's Medical Society was aware of a trademark claim, the designations have been printed in initial capital letters (e.g., Cellex-C).

© 1998 by the People's Medical Society
Printed in the United States of America

Library of Congress Cataloging-in-Publication Data
Hay, Jennifer, 1964–
    Vitamin C : everything you need to know / by Jennifer Hay.
       p. cm.
    Includes index.
    ISBN 1-882606-36-1
      1. Vitamin C—Miscellanea.   2. Vitamin C—Physiological effect.
  I. Title.
QP772.A8H39   1998
612.3'99—dc21   98-10811
                                         CIP

1 2 3 4 5 6 7 8 9 0
First printing, April 1998

CONTENTS

INTRODUCTION

Well, I'm a believer. And I have been for more than 25 years. It was back then that I started taking vitamin C supplements. And I've been taking them ever since.

It all began when I was in my early 20s and found myself getting three or four colds a year. I was eating a healthy diet. And I washed my hands often, especially after being in contact with people who were sick. But try as I might, I was still getting too many colds.

One day, I picked up the newspaper and read an article about Linus Pauling, the eminent chemist and winner of two Nobel Prizes (one in his field, the other for peace). Buried deep in this profile were his thoughts about vitamin C. As you probably know, back then he was the leading, if not the lone, voice on the benefits of using vitamin C supplements. And one of his claims was that vitamin C supplementation could help a person ward off the common cold or lessen its impact if caught early enough.

Hmm, I thought. I need to find out more. So off to the library I went to look up more about Pauling and vitamin C. It didn't take me long to be convinced that it might be worth trying. When I saw how relatively safe vitamin C supplementing was and looked at the research Pauling and others were beginning to release, I figured I would give it a try.

The results were almost miraculous. I started taking 500 milligrams of vitamin C in the morning and before bed. That was in addition to the vitamin C I took in each day through my diet.

For the next two years, I did not get a single cold! Not even a scratchy throat. Just after the second year, I woke up one day feeling a cold coming on. I upped the amount of vitamin C I was taking, and three days later I was symptom-free. This had never happened to me before. My colds had always been long and severe. In the years since then, I have had less than one cold every two years; if I feel one coming on, I up my supplements, and the cold is usually gone in less than a week.

Now, I certainly don't advocate that people follow my regimen, but there's no question that vitamin C supplements have helped me. And from the science that's been emerging in recent years, it seems vitamin C is helping me in other ways.

That is why we have written this book. We all hear and read a lot about vitamin C. But rarely do we find the information all in one place. And even more rarely do we know the reliability of the information. But I can assure you that what you read in this book is reliable and trustworthy. That's because Jennifer Hay, this book's author, has scoured the scientific literature to find the answers. What you will be reading in these pages is not based on our opinion. It comes from sound medical studies and experts in the field. That's why my story is in the introduction, not the main body of this book. My experience is interesting and may be valid, but it is certainly not an expert scientific finding.

Like all other People's Medical Society books, the intention of this book is to empower you. We give you useful and trustworthy information so that you will be able to make better health care decisions for yourself and your family. That has always been our goal.

Each year, we are learning more and more about the effects and benefits of vitamins and minerals. We are confident that this book will help you to be more aware and attuned to these important advances.

CHARLES B. INLANDER
President
People's Medical Society

VITAMIN C

**Everything
You Need
to Know**

Terms printed in boldface can be found in the glossary, beginning on page 113. Only the first mention of the word in the text will be boldfaced.

We have tried to use male and female pronouns in an egalitarian manner throughout the book. Any imbalance in usage has been in the interest of readability.

1 THE BASICS

Q: What is **vitamin C?**

A: Vitamin C, also known as **ascorbic acid** or **ascorbate**, is a white powder that dissolves easily in water. The most well-known of all the **vitamins**, vitamin C is **water soluble**, meaning that it stays in the body only for a short period of time. This means it must be replenished regularly. And countless people do just that. In fact, more people in the United States take vitamin C **supplements** than supplements of any other **nutrient**.

Q: Why is vitamin C so popular?

A: Much of the credit goes to the late Linus Pauling, Ph.D., a Nobel Prize-winning scientist who claimed that vitamin C is effective in preventing colds and treating cancer. Pauling's 1970 book *Vitamin C and the Common Cold* as well as his subsequent publications on vitamin C and cancer caught the attention of the public and of the scientific community, triggering an increase in vitamin C consumption and a good deal of controversy.

Q: **What kind of controversy?**

A: Controversy about whether vitamin C can indeed prevent colds and treat cancer and controversy over the large doses of vitamin C that Pauling said were necessary to achieve those goals.

The popularity and controversy continue today, fed by often-conflicting research that has linked vitamin C to a variety of health benefits, including cancer prevention, heart protection and improved immune response. We discuss this research in the next chapter.

Q: **Does vitamin C play any uncontested roles in the body?**

A: Yes. While vitamin C may be best known for its alleged ability to prevent colds, it plays an undisputed but important role in a number of body functions.

"Since the isolation of ascorbate (vitamin C) from cabbages, oranges and adrenal glands . . . in 1928, this low-molecular mass, water-soluble white crystalline solid has been hailed as the cure for cancer and the common cold. At the other extreme, it has been dismissed as a nutritional hoax, supplements of which are peddled by unscrupulous vitamin manufacturers. As ever, the truth lies somewhere between these extremes."

—Barry Halliwell
American Journal of Clinical Nutrition, June 1997

Q: Such as?

A: Vitamin C is essential for the production of **collagen**, a protein found in connective tissue, cartilage and bone. Collagen acts as a biological cement, holding cells together; it helps support and maintain the structure of tissues, including skin, muscles, gums, blood vessels and bone. Because vitamin C is needed for collagen production, it is essential for the growth and repair of tissues in all parts of the body.

Q: What other roles does it play?

A: Vitamin C helps us metabolize **amino acids**, compounds that form the building blocks of proteins and are, thus, essential to life and health.

Some amino acids are also involved in forming neurotransmitters (chemicals that assist in sending signals among nerve cells in the brain) and hormones (chemicals that regulate the activity of specific organs or groups of cells). Vitamin C contributes to the formation of one of these amino acids—**tyrosine**—which, in turn, contributes to the formation of **epinephrine** and **norepinephrine**. These hormones, which also function as neurotransmitters, help our bodies respond to stress. Researchers believe that vitamin C may also be associated with the release of these hormones from the adrenal glands: Stores of vitamin C in the adrenal glands are depleted when these hormones are mobilized during times of stress.

Vitamin C also plays a role in converting the amino acid **tryptophan** into the neurotransmitter **serotonin**, which controls states of consciousness, mood, sleep and sensitivity to pain.

Q: Anything else?

A: Yes. Vitamin C appears to be necessary for the proper functioning of the **immune system**. It is present in white blood cells, and its ingestion affects levels of a number of substances that regulate the immune system.

Vitamin C also appears to help us metabolize **cholesterol**, folic acid and iron. Vitamin C helps us break down cholesterol so our bodies can dispose of the excess; it plays a role in converting folic acid, a B vitamin, into its biologically active form; and it helps our bodies absorb and use iron. Some research indicates that vitamin C may also help regenerate vitamin E after it has performed its **antioxidant** function. And vitamin C is itself an antioxidant. In fact, it is the body's most powerful water-soluble antioxidant.

Q: I've heard that term a lot recently. What exactly is an antioxidant?

A: An antioxidant is a substance that inhibits oxidative reactions.

Q: OK, but I'm still in the dark about what antioxidants do and why they're important. Could you explain further?

A: Of course. To understand the function of antioxidants, you need to know a little bit about **oxidation**, a chemical process in which a molecule combines with oxygen and loses electrons.

You may recall from chemistry class that atoms contain a nucleus of protons and neutrons surrounded by electrons. These negatively charged electrons generally move in pairs.

Occasionally, however, an atom or molecule contains one or more unpaired electrons. These "lone wolf" particles, known as **free radicals**, make the atom or molecule reactive. Because they lack electrons, atoms or molecules containing free radicals attempt to steal electrons from other molecules to regain their balance. Any molecule victimized by a free radical itself becomes a free radical, initiating a chain reaction of multiplying free radicals.

Q: **What do these free radicals do?**

A: Free radicals can destroy enzymes, protein molecules and even cells. They can interfere with a cell's ability to take in nutrients and expel waste, affecting its ability to perform its functions. They can also damage a cell's genetic material, causing mutations that may lead to cancer. And they can damage fat compounds in the body, causing them to turn rancid and release more free radicals. This process is thought to play a role in cardiovascular disease. In fact, free radicals have been implicated in a variety of diseases as well as the aging process.

Q: **You said these free radicals are created when molecules combine with oxygen. When does this occur?**

A: Oxidative reactions take place in our bodies all the time. We use oxygen for a variety of cellular activities—from generating energy to manufacturing enzymes. The very cellular activities that keep us alive involve oxidation and the production of free radicals. In fact, cells in our immune system deliberately make free radicals to kill bacteria, viruses and other harmful foreign organisms.

Exposure to substances in our environment—ultraviolet light, cigarette smoke and pollutants, for example—can also trigger the production of free radicals.

Q: OK. I think I've got the idea. Now could you tell me again where antioxidants fit in?

A: Certainly. Antioxidants, as we've said, are substances that inhibit oxidative reactions. They offer electrons to free radicals, thus neutralizing them. This gesture stops the free radical chain reaction and renders the antioxidant inactive.

Q: How does all this relate to vitamin C?

A: Vitamin C is an antioxidant. It has been shown in test-tube studies to stop oxidative chain reactions. Many researchers theorize that vitamin C and other antioxidant nutrients may help protect us from the damage caused by free radicals, which, as we've said, have been implicated in a number of diseases.

Other nutrients that act as antioxidants include vitamin E, beta carotene and the **mineral** selenium.

Q: I have a general understanding of what vitamins and minerals are, but I don't really know the difference between them. What are the basic definitions?

A: Vitamins and minerals are nutrients—food components obtained from our diets—that have been found to be essential in small quantities for human life. Vitamins are organic compounds; this means that they contain carbon and come from living materials—plants or animals—or from substances derived from living materials, such as petroleum products. Minerals, in contrast, are inorganic compounds; they do not contain carbon and do not originate from living organisms.

Q: So vitamin C is organic. Do we make it ourselves?

A: While plants and most animals are able to make their own vitamin C, fruit bats, guinea pigs and primates—including humans—are not. We are missing an enzyme crucial to the manufacture of the vitamin, so we must obtain it from our diet.

Q: From orange juice, right?

A: That's one source, yes. A number of fruits and vegetables are rich in vitamin C. In addition to such well-known sources as oranges, grapefruits and other citrus fruits, vitamin C is found in strawberries, kiwifruits, black currants, guavas, papayas, cantaloupes and tomatoes. Vegetables also offer a healthy share; good sources include bell peppers, broccoli, brussels sprouts, cabbages, peas, potatoes, asparagus and dark green leafy vegetables.

> *Among the more exotic sources of vitamin C are cactus pads, celeriac, cherimoya, jicama, longan, litchi nuts, salsify, seaweed and tamarillos.*

Q: How much vitamin C do we need?

A: The **Recommended Dietary Allowance (RDA)**, the amount that the National Academy of Sciences' Food and Nutrition Board considers to be adequate to meet the known nutrient needs of most healthy individuals, is 60 milligrams. The RDA for smokers is higher—100 milligrams—because cigarette smoking is known to deplete the body's supply of vitamin C.

Q: But aren't the amounts in most supplements a lot higher?

A: Yes. While some multivitamin supplements provide only the RDA, other multivitamin supplements, as well as individual supplements, provide vitamin C in amounts substantially higher than the RDA.

Q: Why is that?

A: The RDAs as they currently exist are designed to meet our known nutrient needs—they are the amounts we need to prevent deficiency diseases. But much of the research into vitamin C indicates that amounts above the RDA may be needed for optimal health.

Q: Do we know what those amounts are?

A: Not yet, but the experts are working on it. The varying amounts used in studies of vitamin C's effect on a multitude of medical conditions provide us with clues. So do studies that measure the direct effects that varying amounts of vitamin C have on the body. The Food and Nutrition Board will likely take this research into account in its systematic review and update of the RDAs.

In fact, this process is now underway. The first of the new **Dietary Reference Intakes (DRIs)** was introduced in August 1997. These guidelines, which will be introduced sporadically from now through the year 2000, place more emphasis on the benefits people can derive from nutrients than do the existing RDAs. The DRIs include revised RDAs designed not only to prevent deficiency diseases but also to decrease the risk of chronic diseases such as cancer, heart disease and osteoporosis. The new RDAs are based in part on the Estimated Average Requirement, an amount that meets the estimated nutrient need of half the individuals in a specific group. When not enough information is available to estimate an average requirement, the DRIs establish an Adequate Intake, an amount that appears to sustain a desired indicator of health, such as calcium retention in bone. The DRIs also include a Tolerable Upper Intake Level, the maximum amount unlikely to cause side effects in most healthy people.

> *The following vegetables provide 100 percent or more of the RDA for vitamin C in a single, 3½ ounce serving: arugula, broccoli, brussels sprouts, cauliflower, fennel, kale, mustard greens, peppers and turnip greens.*

Q: **Will the new DRIs indicate a higher intake of vitamin C?**

A: That remains to be seen; however, many of the studies that have shown health benefits from vitamin C have involved doses well in excess of the RDA.

Q: Are there any side effects associated with high doses of vitamin C?

A: Vitamin C is considered relatively safe even in large amounts because excess amounts are excreted in the urine. Doses of 500 milligrams or more have been known to cause diarrhea in some people, but many people can take much larger doses with no problems. Large doses of vitamin C have also been linked to kidney stones, although this link is somewhat controversial. We discuss dosage and side effects in more detail in chapter 3.

Q: What happens when we don't get enough vitamin C?

A: Mild deficiencies can result in easy bruising (caused by fragile capillaries), delayed wound healing and reduced resistance to infections. Serious deficiencies can result in **scurvy**, which is associated with bleeding gums, loose teeth, joint tenderness and swelling, extreme weakness and fatigue, hemorrhaging under the skin, anemia and poor wound healing.

Q: Is deficiency common?

A: Serious vitamin C deficiencies are not often seen in the United States and other developed countries. A mere 10 milligrams of vitamin C daily—the amount in 3½ table-spoons of orange juice—can prevent scurvy. But that doesn't mean we are getting adequate amounts. Dietary surveys indicate that between 20 and 30 percent of U.S. adults take in less than the RDA. And studies show that certain groups of the population—most notably alcoholics, the critically ill and the institutionalized elderly—are often deficient.

Q: What about sailors? I seem to recall reading somewhere that they don't get enough vitamin C.

A: Historically, scurvy was common among sailors, whose dried-biscuit-and-meat diets were often lacking in vitamin C. In the eighteenth century, however, a British doctor discovered that adding limes to the sailors' rations prevented the dreaded disease. Eventually, the British Navy made it a regular practice to issue daily rations of limes or other citrus fruits to sailors on long sea voyages, earning the sailors the nickname *limey.*

Q: So we've known about vitamin C for more than 200 years?

A: Yes and no. The experiences of the British sailors demonstrated that *something* in citrus is necessary to maintain health. But it was not until the 1930s that that something—vitamin C—was isolated and synthesized. And while research has since shown that vitamin C plays a variety of important roles in the body, we do not yet know the extent of vitamin C's effects on our health. As we've said, some studies have linked vitamin C to such health benefits as heart protection, cancer prevention and improved immunity, while others have failed to find a link. We look at the research into vitamin C's possible health benefits in the next chapter.

2 VITAMIN C AND ITS USES

Q: You said in chapter 1 that vitamin C has been linked to a number of health benefits. What are they?

A: In addition to vitamin C's known bodily functions— helping us to produce collagen, metabolize amino acids, cholesterol and nutrients, and maintain a healthy immune system—it has also been credited with the following:

- protecting against heart disease and **stroke**
- improving **immune response** (including the response to viruses that cause colds)
- protecting against cancer
- protecting the lungs
- protecting against **cataracts**
- protecting the skin
- speeding wound healing
- decreasing diabetic complications
- slowing the progression of **osteoarthritis**
- improving fertility

Q: Can vitamin C really do all that?

A: Maybe, maybe not. Many of the claims made for vitamin C have some substance; they are rooted in scientific theory and supported, at least in part, by research. But the research often conflicts. One well-designed study may show that vitamin C provides a substantial health benefit; the next study on the very same subject may show that the vitamin has no effect. More research is needed. Until a consensus emerges, vitamin C's various health benefits remain a matter of speculation.

Q: Is there any chance vitamin C may do at least some of what it's claimed to do?

A: Yes. The evidence available thus far indicates that vitamin C may indeed play some role in helping our bodies fight disease.

In recent years, researchers have been looking into the possibility that antioxidants may help prevent the degenerative diseases of aging, and some **epidemiologic studies** have linked low intakes or low blood levels of antioxidant nutrients such as vitamin C with increased mortality from chronic diseases.

"There is considerable evidence that a high intake of supplementary ascorbate improves the health and helps to control various diseases."

—Linus Pauling, Ph.D.

Q: I want to know more about these studies, but first could you explain why the researchers look at both intake and blood levels? Wouldn't a low intake automatically result in a low blood level and a high intake automatically result in a high blood level?

A: In most cases, yes. But blood or **plasma** levels of vitamin C—and other nutrients, for that matter—are also affected by a variety of other factors. For example, you may recall from chapter 1 that smokers require more vitamin C than nonsmokers. This is because smoking decreases the blood levels of vitamin C. A smoker and a nonsmoker could take in the same amount of vitamin C, but the smoker will usually have a lower blood level of the vitamin.

Q: Why is that?

A: Because the smoker's body uses more vitamin C than the nonsmoker's body—much in the way an active person's body uses more calories than an inactive person's body.

Q: I see. What other factors affect blood levels of vitamin C?

A: Illness is a major factor; blood levels of vitamin C are generally lower in people who are ill than in people who are healthy, as we discuss later in the chapter. But blood levels of vitamin C can also be affected by dietary and lifestyle factors such as age, body mass and consumption of alcohol, calories and fat as well as tobacco use and vitamin C intake (*American Journal of Clinical Nutrition,* June 1997).

Q: No wonder researchers need to look at both blood levels and intake! Getting back to those studies that link intake or blood levels of vitamin C with mortality from chronic diseases, what exactly do they show?

A: Here's a sampling of some of the findings.

- Researchers at the National Institute on Aging compared the use of vitamin C and vitamin E supplements with death rates in 11,179 older people during a three-year period and found that those who used both supplements were 42 percent less likely to die of any cause and 53 percent less likely to die of heart problems during the study period than were those who used neither supplement. While the use of vitamin C supplements alone did not significantly reduce the risk of death, the use of both vitamin C and E supplements conferred more protection than did the use of vitamin E supplements alone (*American Journal of Clinical Nutrition*, August 1996).

- Tufts University researchers who followed 747 older people for nine to 12 years found that those with higher plasma levels of vitamin C were between 36 and 46 percent less likely to die of any cause during the period than were those with lower levels. The decreased risk was attributed primarily to a decrease in deaths due to heart problems (*American Journal of Epidemiology*, September 1996).

- A study reported in the May 1992 *Epidemiology* examined the relation between vitamin C intake and mortality in 11,348 adults and found that men with the highest vitamin C intake were 35 percent less likely to die of any cause, 42 percent less likely to die of heart disease and 22 percent less likely to die of cancer during the study period than were men with the lowest vitamin C intake.

VITAMIN C AND THE CARDIOVASCULAR SYSTEM

Q: Those studies seem to imply that vitamin C really does protect against heart disease. What's the story?

A: Vitamin C's association with heart disease, like its association with many other diseases, is still unclear. While some studies—including those we've just summarized—indicate that vitamin C protects the heart and blood vessels, others do not confirm these findings.

The Iowa Women's Health Study, a large study of post-menopausal women, for example, found no association between vitamin C intake and the risk of death from coronary heart disease (*New England Journal of Medicine,* May 2, 1996). And the Nurses' Health Study and the Health Professionals' Follow-up Study, widely publicized studies that pushed vitamin E's heart-protective effects into the spotlight, found no relation between vitamin C intake and rates of heart attack or death from other heart-related problems (*New England Journal of Medicine,* May 20, 1993). Still, other research indicates that vitamin C may play a role in some aspects of cardiovascular health.

"Cardiovascular disease, disease of the heart and blood vessels, constitutes the principal cause of death. During recent years, it has been discovered that nutritional and environmental factors are important in determining the incidence of cardiovascular disease. Some epidemiological evidence . . . indicates that vitamin C is the most important of these factors."

—Ewan Cameron, M.D., and Linus Pauling, Ph.D.
Cancer and Vitamin C, 1979

Q: Which aspects?

A: Vitamin C's role in collagen production helps maintain the integrity of blood vessels, which, in turn, helps keep the vessels—the vascular part of the cardiovascular system—in proper working order.

Vitamin C also plays a role in metabolizing cholesterol. High levels of cholesterol in the blood have been linked to the development of **atherosclerosis**, a buildup of **plaque**, or fatty deposits, on artery walls that contributes to **coronary-artery disease** and stroke. There is some evidence that vitamin C may help keep cholesterol levels in check. In addition, some studies indicate that vitamin C may help lower blood pressure and influence blood's tendency to clot.

Vitamin C and Cholesterol

Q: You've said that vitamin C helps us metabolize cholesterol. In what way?

A: Vitamin C is needed to convert cholesterol into **bile acids**. Bile acids are the primary way in which excess cholesterol is eliminated from the body. Without adequate vitamin C intake, the body cannot effectively eliminate excess cholesterol, which, theoretically, can result in high serum, or blood, cholesterol levels.

> *The albedo—the white membrane under the skin of an orange—is richer in vitamin C than the fruit itself; it is also rich in pectin, a type of soluble fiber thought to help lower cholesterol levels.*

Q: Is that how vitamin C is thought to keep cholesterol levels in check, by enabling us to get rid of the excess?

A: It's one way, yes. Some studies have shown that high serum cholesterol levels decrease when people are given vitamin C supplements, and people with low vitamin C intakes are often found to have high serum cholesterol levels. In one of the newer studies on the subject, researchers found that while vitamin C intake had no relation to cholesterol levels in girls with normal cholesterol levels, it decreased total serum cholesterol levels in girls with levels above 200 milligrams per deciliter (mg/dL). Each 100-milligram-per-day increase in dietary vitamin C was associated with a decrease of between 4 and 13 mg/dL (*Epidemiology*, November 1993).

Q: Does vitamin C have any other effect on cholesterol levels?

A: Vitamin C may have a positive effect on the ratio between **high-density lipoprotein (HDL)**, the so-called good cholesterol, and **low-density lipoprotein (LDL)**, the so-called bad cholesterol, as well as an effect on the level of **triglycerides**, other fatty compounds found in the blood. Some studies indicate that increasing vitamin C intake—with either supplements or food—may increase HDL levels and decrease LDL and/or triglyceride levels, although other studies have failed to find such an effect.

Q: What, specifically, did the studies supporting vitamin C's positive effect on HDL, LDL and triglyceride levels find?

A: The answer depends on the study.

- Researchers at Tufts University in Boston found that vitamin C in excess of the RDA lowers LDL levels and raises HDL levels. In women, HDL levels peaked when blood levels of vitamin C reached 1 mg/dL. In men, HDL levels continued to rise parallel with vitamin C blood levels, while LDL dropped significantly.

- The Baltimore Longitudinal Study of Aging and a 1994 study by U.S. Department of Agriculture and National Institute of Health researchers both found that high levels of vitamin C in the blood correspond with higher levels of HDL.

- A study published in the November 1996 *European Journal of Clinical Nutrition* found that eating a lot of vitamin-C rich foods increases serum HDL and lowers serum triglycerides.

Q: Interesting. But didn't you say that other studies have failed to find a link?

A: Yes. Another Tufts University study, published in the January 1995 *Annals of Epidemiology,* found that vitamin C supplementation of 1,000 milligrams (1 gram) per day for eight months had no significant effect on HDL, LDL, total cholesterol or triglyceride levels.

Vitamin C supplementation did, however, increase HDL levels in a subgroup of study participants who had low blood levels of vitamin C at the beginning of the study.

Q: It sounds like vitamin C does have some sort of effect on cholesterol levels. But what exactly do cholesterol levels have to do with heart disease?

A: High total cholesterol levels and high LDL cholesterol levels increase the risk of atherosclerosis and coronary-artery disease, while high HDL cholesterol levels decrease the risk.

Q: Why is that?

A: Excess LDL cholesterol tends to stick to artery walls, contributing to the buildup of plaque, while HDL helps remove excess cholesterol from the body.

Q: What exactly happens when LDL sticks to artery walls?

A: The most widely held theory takes us back to our discussion of oxidation. LDL cholesterol tends to stick in places where the innermost layer of cells—the **endothelium**—has been damaged. Once there, many researchers believe, it squeezes through the spaces between the endothelial cells until it is inside the wall of the artery. There, it reacts with oxygen, creating potentially harmful free radicals. This process, known as **lipid peroxidation**, sets off a chain reaction that attracts more LDL cholesterol, creates more free radicals and results in the buildup of plaque, which narrows the arteries.

Q: Can vitamin C do anything to prevent this chain reaction?

A: Perhaps. Some researchers believe that vitamin C may help prevent LDL from oxidizing or at least stop the oxidative chain reaction. It may do this directly, by acting as an antioxidant, or indirectly, by returning vitamin E to its active antioxidant stage.

Q: Is there any indication that vitamin C actually does this?

A: Yes. Vitamin C has been shown in some test-tube studies to inhibit LDL oxidation. In fact, it is the first of the antioxidants present in plasma to be used up when lipids such as LDL are oxidized. Because lipid peroxidation is detectable only after all of the vitamin C in plasma has been used up, some researchers have speculated that it is the only antioxidant that can actually prevent lipid peroxidation.

Q: That's all well and good, but my arteries aren't test tubes. Have any studies looked at vitamin C's direct effect on atherosclerosis in animals or people?

A: Yes on both counts. Large doses of vitamin C have been shown to slow the progression of atherosclerosis in rabbits. The results of human studies have not been as promising, however. One recent study of men with coronary-artery disease looked at the effect of vitamin C and vitamin E supplementation on the progression of atherosclerosis and found that vitamin C supplements had no effect on progression when given alone or in conjunction with vitamin E (*Journal of the American Medical Association,* June 21, 1995).

Q: So what's the bottom line?

A: The bottom line is that while vitamin C may be capable of preventing LDL from oxidizing, it may not have a direct effect on plaque buildup. This does not mean, however, that it has no effect on either atherosclerosis or coronary-artery disease.

As we've seen, vitamin C does appear to affect cholesterol levels, and high cholesterol levels are risk factors for atherosclerosis and coronary-artery disease. And as Boston University School of Medicine researchers point out in a review article on the role of antioxidants in atherosclerotic heart disease, coronary-artery disease involves more than just the development of plaque. It also involves the rupture of plaque, constriction of blood vessels and formation of clots. The researchers note that antioxidants may stabilize plaque so it won't rupture, protect the blood vessel walls and prevent **platelets,** small, disk-shaped structures in the blood, from clumping together to form clots (*New England Journal of Medicine,* August 7, 1997).

Vitamin C and Blood Pressure

Q: Didn't you say vitamin C may also help lower blood pressure?

A: Yes. Several studies have identified a link between **hypertension,** or high blood pressure, and vitamin C. And although the evidence is not conclusive, there is some indication that vitamin C can help lower blood pressure.

Q: What is the link?

A: People with low vitamin C intake or low levels of vitamin C in their blood appear to be at increased risk for hypertension.

- A 1984 study reported in the *International Journal of Vitamin Nutrition Research* found a correlation between blood levels of vitamin C and systolic blood pressure (the upper number in a blood pressure reading) in 194 people between the ages of 30 and 39. Those with higher levels of vitamin C in their blood were less likely to have high systolic blood pressure than were those with lower levels.

- A 1988 study reported in the *American Journal of Clinical Nutrition* found an association between low plasma levels of vitamin C and raised blood pressure in men with high blood pressure.

- Researchers examining the relationship between vitamin C deficiency and heart attack found that vitamin C deficiency was associated with high blood pressure (*British Medical Journal,* March 1, 1995).

Q: What about the evidence that vitamin C may actually lower blood pressure?

A: Several studies show that vitamin C supplementation has a modest effect on blood pressure levels.

- In a small study of 40 middle-aged men who were given either vitamin C supplements or **placebo**, or inactive, pills, systolic blood pressure decreased by 2.5 mm Hg (millimeter of Mercury) in those who received the supplements and by only 0.2 mm Hg in those who received the placebo (*Life Chemistry Reports,* 1994).

- A study published in the *Journal of Human Hypertension* (August 1993) found that older people given 400 milligrams of vitamin C per day for four weeks saw a 3 mm Hg decrease in their systolic pressure and a 0.4 mm Hg decrease in their diastolic blood pressure (the lower number in a blood pressure reading) compared with older people who took placebos.

- British researchers reported in a 1994 issue of *Gerontology* that older people given 500 milligrams of vitamin C for six weeks saw their systolic blood pressure drop 2.6 mm Hg and their diastolic blood pressure drop 1.2 mm Hg compared with older people who were given placebos.

Q: Those study results seem to confirm one another. Why did you say the evidence that vitamin C can help lower blood pressure is inconclusive?

A: Because not all studies have produced similar results. A study reported in the January 1994 *Age and Ageing,* for example, found that while blood pressure was higher in older people with low dietary intake of antioxidants, vitamin C supplements were no more likely to lower blood pressure than were placebos.

Q: So, what's a person to believe? Does vitamin C lower blood pressure or doesn't it?

A: There is as yet no definitive answer. Still, in an editorial about research on vitamin C's effects on heart disease and stroke, Christopher J. Bulpitt, M.D., a professor of geriatric medicine at Royal Postgraduate Medical School in London, states that "vitamin C probably does lower blood pressure" (*British Medical Journal,* June 17, 1995).

As the studies show, however, the reduction is small. Bulpitt notes that vitamin C's effect on blood pressure may not be sufficient to have a significant effect on heart disease or stroke.

Vitamin C and Other Factors

Q: Well, then, does vitamin C do anything else that might protect the heart and blood vessels?

A: It appears so. Recent studies indicate that vitamin C may help dilate blood vessels and prevent blood from clotting, both of which can reduce the risk of heart attacks. In fact, a study published in the March 1, 1997, *British Medical Journal* found that middle-aged men with low blood levels of vitamin C have more than twice the risk of heart attack as middle-aged men with adequate blood levels of vitamin C.

Q: Can vitamin C actually be used to prevent heart attacks?

A: Possibly. Several studies indicate that vitamin C may be beneficial for people with coronary-artery disease— people who are at high risk for heart attacks.

• People with blocked arteries showed a marked improvement in the dilation of their brachial arteries (the arteries that run down the length of the arms) when they were given 2,000 milligrams (2 grams) of vitamin C. Before they were given vitamin C, their arteries opened only 2 percent when the demand for blood increased during a testing situation. After they were given vitamin C, their arteries opened nearly 10 percent—an increase that wasn't observed in patients who were given placebos (*Circulation,* March 15, 1996).

- In two separate studies, researchers at the University of Freiburg in Germany reported that vitamin C improved the effectiveness of vessel-dilating drugs in people with coronary-artery disease and in smokers, who are at greater risk of coronary-artery disease. Vessel-dilating drugs, known as **vasodilators**, are often prescribed to people with coronary-artery disease to help stave off heart attacks.

- Japanese researchers studied 119 patients with heart disease who underwent **angioplasty** (a procedure in which a balloon is inserted through a narrowed artery, then inflated to widen the artery) and found that only 24 percent of those who took 500 milligrams of vitamin C each day in the four months after surgery developed new artery blockages compared with 43 percent of the patients who did not take vitamin C (*Journal of the American College of Cardiology,* December 1, 1996).

- A study reported in the June 17, 1995, *British Medical Journal* concluded that a 60-milligram-per-day increase in vitamin C—the amount in one orange—might reduce the risk of heart attack by 10 percent in people who take in approximately the RDA.

Q: How can the equivalent of only one orange a day reduce heart attack risk?

A: The researchers found that even modest increases in vitamin C intake may be able to decrease the formation of blood clots. And clots, as you probably know, can block the arteries leading to the heart, depriving the heart of oxygen and damaging the heart muscle; in other words, clots can cause heart attacks.

Q: How might vitamin C prevent clots from forming?

A: The researchers found that increases in vitamin C intake decrease the amount of **fibrinogen** in the blood. Fibrinogen is a blood component that plays a role in blood clotting.

Q: Have any other studies linked vitamin C intake to a decrease in blood clotting?

A: Yes. In one study, postsurgical patients given 1,000 milligrams (1 gram) of vitamin C a day developed fewer life-threatening blood clots than did those who did not get vitamin C.

Q: What about people who have had heart attacks? Can vitamin C do anything for them?

A: Possibly. According to a study reported in the July 1995 *Journal of the American Dietetic Association,* heart attack survivors who ate fruits and vegetables high in vitamin C in the 10 days after their attacks had lower blood levels of an enzyme that indicates the degree of heart damage than did heart attack survivors who ate little vitamin C. The researchers theorize that free radicals released during the heart attack stay in the heart and continue to damage the muscle if vitamin C isn't there to dispose of them.

Q: **Wow. Sounds like vitamin C is covering all—or at least most—of the bases. Does it do anything else that may protect the heart and blood vessels?**

A: Yes. As we mentioned earlier, the oxidation of LDL cholesterol is not the sole means by which arteries become clogged. Nor is the prevention of LDL oxidation the only means by which vitamin C may slow the progression of atherosclerosis or coronary-artery disease.

In 1990, researchers at Vanderbilt University in Nashville discovered a class of chemicals known as F2-isoprostanes. These chemicals are produced by the oxidation of fats in the body and are thought to contribute to the development of plaque, particularly in cigarette smokers, who produce more of the chemicals than do nonsmokers. According to researchers at the University of Pennsylvania in Philadelphia, vitamin C supplements may help decrease levels of these potentially harmful chemicals. When the researchers gave 2,000 milligrams (2 grams) of vitamin C a day to smokers for five days, the levels of one isoprostane in the smokers dropped significantly (*Circulation,* July 1, 1996).

Another factor that may contribute to atherosclerosis is the tendency of white blood cells known as **leukocytes** to stick to the endothelium, the smooth tissue that lines blood vessels. This tendency is particularly prominent among smokers. Vitamin C may help reduce this tendency—at least that's what animal studies have shown. Researchers gave vitamin C to hamsters—either as part of the diet or intravenously—and then exposed them to cigarette smoke. The vitamin appeared to offer protection to the rodents, reducing their leukocytes' tendency to stick to blood vessel walls (*Proceedings of the National Academy of Sciences,* August 2, 1994).

Vitamin C and Stroke

Q: Didn't you say that atherosclerosis also contributes to stroke? Does vitamin C have any effect on stroke risk?

A: Yes on both counts. Many of the risk factors for heart disease—atherosclerosis, high blood pressure and high cholesterol, for example—are also risk factors for stroke—as is heart disease itself. Consequently, any effect vitamin C has on these risk factors is likely to translate into an effect on stroke risk.

Q: I take it the effect is a beneficial one?

A: It certainly is. Studies in Switzerland, Norway, the United Kingdom and the United States have associated low intakes or blood levels of vitamin C with increased risk of stroke. And several recent studies indicate that higher vitamin C intakes or blood levels may confer some protection.

- The Western Electric Study monitored the health and dietary habits of 1,843 American men for 30 years and found that those who consumed the most vitamin C were 29 percent less likely to have strokes than were those who consumed the least amount of vitamin C (*Nutrition Research Newsletter,* June 1997).

- British researchers followed 730 elderly men and women for 20 years and found that those who consumed the most vitamin C were 60 percent less likely to die of stroke than were those who consumed the least. Incidentally, most of their vitamin C intake came from foods (*British Medical Journal,* June 17, 1995).

Q: Whew! That's a lot to digest. Before we go on, could you summarize how vitamin C might help protect the heart and blood vessels?

A: Certainly. Some studies indicate that vitamin C may protect the heart and blood vessels by doing the following:

- maintaining the integrity of blood vessels

- helping to eliminate excess cholesterol

- increasing levels of HDL, or good, cholesterol

- decreasing levels of LDL, or bad, cholesterol

- preventing LDL cholesterol from oxidizing or stopping the oxidative chain reaction

- lowering blood pressure

- helping blood vessels dilate

- reducing the risk of blood clotting

VITAMIN C AND THE IMMUNE SYSTEM

Q: You've said that vitamin C is necessary for the immune system to function properly. Is this how it protects against other diseases?

A: It's one way, yes. The immune system is our body's system of defense against bacteria, viruses and other harmful invaders that cause disease—including infections and cancer.

Q: What parts of the body play a role in the immune system?

A: The major components of the immune system include the bone marrow and **thymus** gland, which manufacture and process white blood cells; the tissues, vessels, organs and nodes of the lymphatic system, which filters and conveys a fluid known as lymph and produces various types of white blood cells; and the white blood cells themselves. These cells, known as leukocytes, are present throughout the body in blood and lymph and play an important role in fending off foreign substances.

Q: What do these blood cells do?

A: That depends on the type of cell. There are several different kinds of leukocytes, and each plays a different role in the immune response.

B lymphocytes, or B cells, are responsible for a type of immune response known as **humoral immunity**. They identify potentially harmful foreign substances and attempt to render them harmless. They do this by producing **antibodies**, which attach to the substance and neutralize it much in the way antioxidants neutralize free radicals.

T lymphocytes, or T cells, initiate, direct and terminate a type of immune response known as **cell-mediated immunity**. They stimulate B cells to produce antibodies and to attack and kill invaders within specific cells. T cells also destroy invaders directly and produce chemicals called **lymphokines**, which stimulate **phagocytes** to attack and kill invaders.

Phagocytes are cells that engulf, or ingest, bacteria, viruses, cell fragments and abnormal cells such as those that lead to cancer.

Q: That sounds like quite an army. Are any other troops involved?

A: Yes. Other chemicals are also crucial to the function of the immune system. These chemicals, known as **mediators**, are released from cells when foreign substances meet up with antibodies or T cells. Their release can trigger a variety of bodily reactions, including inflammation, changes in blood pressure and dilation or contraction of blood vessels.

Q: How does vitamin C come into play in all this?

A: Vitamin C appears to play a role in the functioning of the thymus gland, which, as you recall, manufactures and processes white blood cells. Large amounts of vitamin C have been shown in studies to stimulate the production of T cells and B cells.

Q: Didn't you say that vitamin C is actually present in the white blood cells?

A: Yes, we did. And levels of vitamin C in these cells drop when the body is fighting an infection or chronic illness.

Q: Is that why we're often told to increase our intake of vitamin C when we're sick?

A: Yes.

Q: Does the level of vitamin C in our bodies have any other effect on our immune system?

A: Yes. Vitamin C levels also affect the levels of a number of important mediators, those chemicals released when our immune system encounters a foreign substance.

Q: Are there any other connections between vitamin C and the immune system?

A: An indirect one, yes. Vitamin C is thought to protect the body from the damage inflicted by the immune system itself. As we noted in chapter 1, the immune response involves oxidation. Free radicals are generated when the white blood cells fight bacteria, viruses and other microorganisms. Vitamin C is thought to protect the immune system and other parts of the body from any damage caused by these oxidative reactions.

Vitamin C and Immune Response

Q: You've used that term "immune response" before. What exactly does it mean?

A: Immune response is the body's defense against invading antigens and cancer—in other words, the way the immune system functions. We outlined the two types of immune response—humoral and cell-mediated immunity—in our discussion of the roles played by the various parts of the immune system.

> *"There is much evidence that vitamin C is essential for the efficient working of the immune system. . . . The simplest and safest way to enhance immunocompetence in these patients and to ensure that their molecular and cell-mediated defense systems are working at maximum efficiency is to increase their intake of vitamin C."*
>
> —Ewan Cameron, M.D., and Linus Pauling, Ph.D.
> *Cancer and Vitamin C*, 1979

Q: That clears things up a bit. Now, is there any connection between vitamin C and immune response?

A: Yes. As we've said, the amount of vitamin C present in the blood—and in the white blood cells themselves—drops when the body is fighting an infection or chronic illness, which indicates that vitamin C plays a role in immune response. In addition, there is evidence that increased intake of vitamin C during infections and chronic illnesses may lessen their severity and/or help speed recovery.

Q: I'd like to know more. Have any studies actually looked at the association between vitamin C and illness?

A: Yes. Studies show that people with infections and other illnesses have lower blood levels of vitamin C than healthy individuals, and the sicker they are, the lower their vitamin C levels.

British researchers who tested the blood of critically ill patients found that the levels of vitamin C in their plasma were less than 25 percent of those of healthy people and that levels were lowest in the sickest individuals (*American Journal of Clinical Nutrition,* May 1996). These findings correspond with those of two other studies of vitamin C levels in the critically ill.

But the critically ill may benefit from vitamin C supplementation. In a 1984 study, critically ill elderly patients given 200 milligrams of vitamin C a day had higher levels of vitamin C in their white blood cells than similar people given a placebo. Those with higher vitamin C levels in their blood cells were less likely to die of their illnesses than were those with lower levels; they also took less time to recover from their illnesses.

Q: **What about healthy people? Is there any evidence that vitamin C boosts their immune response?**

A: Yes. Several recent studies have found that immune responses improve when healthy people take in more than the RDA of vitamin C, vitamin E or beta carotene.

- One study showed that immune function as measured by delayed hypersensitivity skin tests decreased when the vitamin C intake of healthy men was reduced from 250 to 5, 10 or 20 milligrams per day for 60 days. During these tests, the men were injected with small amounts of different **antigens**—substances that could cause infection or disease. When the immune system is functioning well, it produces antibodies to protect the body from the antigens and the infections or diseases they cause. The production of these antibodies produces a visible skin reaction that indicates the immune system is functioning well. In this study, the number of reactions the men experienced decreased as their vitamin intake decreased.

- In a study reported in the September 1994 *American Journal of Clinical Nutrition,* the number of reactions to delayed sensitivity skin tests increased in healthy older people who took a standard multivitamin supplement—including 90 milligrams of vitamin C—once a day for a year.

Vitamin C and Cancer

Q: **I thought vitamin C's antioxidant role was responsible for cancer protection. Why are we discussing it now?**

A: Because vitamin C's role in the immune system is also thought to confer some protection against cancer.

Q: **No wonder vitamin C's link to cancer is such a hot topic! But didn't you say vitamin C's protective effects in this regard are somewhat controversial?**

A: Yes. While vitamin C's ability to protect against cancer is theoretically possible, claims that it can cure or treat cancer have not been substantiated.

"It is our opinion that supplemental vitamin C is of some benefit to patients with all forms of cancer, and it is our belief that, in time, this simple and safe form of supportive treatment will become an accepted part of all regimes for the treatment of cancer."
—Ewan Cameron, M.D., and Linus Pauling, Ph.D.
International Journal of Environmental Studies, 1977

Q: What about prevention? Can vitamin C help prevent cancer?

A: Perhaps. Substantial evidence indicates that a diet high in fruits and vegetables—foods that are rich in vitamin C—helps prevent cancer, but studies attempting to link vitamin C directly to reduced cancer risk have produced conflicting results.

Vitamin C and Cancer Prevention

Q: I'd like to know more. Could we start with the studies about fruits and vegetables?

A: Certainly. More than 100 epidemiological studies have found that people who eat diets rich in fruits and vegetables—foods that are rich in vitamin C—are less likely to develop cancer than those who eat few fruits and vegetables. In fact, these studies indicate that a diet rich in fruit and vegetables (five or more servings a day) cuts the risk of some cancers—notably those of the gastrointestinal tract and the lungs—nearly in half.

Because people who eat a lot of fruits and vegetables generally take in more vitamin C than those who eat few fruits and vegetables, many people have theorized that vitamin C, with its antioxidant power, may be responsible for this protective effect. Indeed, many studies have shown that people with higher intakes of vitamin C—particularly vitamin C obtained from dietary sources—are at reduced risk of cancer. But other studies have failed to find a connection between vitamin C intake and cancer.

Q: Does cancer location have anything to do with the conflicting results?

A: Apparently not, as the following pairs of studies indicate.

- A recent study conducted by researchers at the National Cancer Institute compared the diets of 10,000 Americans with their incidence of lung cancer over a 19-year period and found that those who took in the most vitamin C were 44 percent less likely to develop lung cancer than those who took in the least (*American Journal of Epidemiology,* August 1, 1997). A similar study of Finnish men and women, published in the same issue of the journal, however, found that vitamin C had no effect on the incidence of lung cancer.

- Italian researchers who compared the dietary intakes of some 1,200 individuals with colon or rectal cancer with the dietary intakes of approximately 2,000 similar individuals without cancer found that those who took in the most vitamin C were 60 percent less likely to develop cancer than those with the lowest intake (*British Journal of Cancer,* December 1994). But in a study reported in the July 21, 1994, *New England Journal of Medicine,* vitamin C supplements did not reduce the development of colorectal **polyps,** growths that are precursors of colorectal cancer. In this widely publicized study, 864 adults were randomly assigned to receive a placebo; 25 milligrams per day of beta carotene; 1,000 milligrams (1 gram) of vitamin C and 400 milligrams of vitamin E per day; or a combination of vitamins C and E and beta carotene. During the four years of the study, those given vitamins C and E actually were 8 percent more likely to develop polyps than those given the placebo. Adding to the confusion,

a study reported in the December 1, 1996, *American
Journal of Epidemiology* failed to find a link between
vitamin C intake and a reduction in polyp incidence in
men but did find a link in women.

• State University of New York researchers who looked
at the diets of 297 premenopausal women with breast
cancer and 311 healthy premenopausal women found
that the women whose diets included the most vitamin
C were 47 percent less likely to develop breast cancer
than were women whose diets included the least
amount of vitamin C; the researchers found no relationship between breast cancer risk and vitamin C supplements, however (*Journal of the National Cancer
Institute,* March 20, 1996). Similar results have been
observed in postmenopausal women. The Netherlands
Cohort Study, which followed 62,000 postmenopausal
for more than four years, found that while vitamin C
supplements had no effect on the incidence of breast
cancer, dietary intake of vitamin C appeared to confer
some protection. Women who took in the highest
amount of dietary vitamin C were 33 percent less likely
to develop breast cancer than were women who took
in the lowest amounts (*British Journal of Cancer:
Breast Cancer,* January 1997).

Q: OK. I get the picture. But before we go on, could
you tell me what other types of cancers have
been studied in connection with vitamin C?

A: In addition to lung cancer, colorectal cancer and breast
cancer, researchers have studied vitamin C's effects on
stomach, esophageal, bladder, cervical and prostate cancer.
    In general, more studies indicate that vitamin C has a pro-
tective effect against stomach, esophageal and lung cancer than

indicate protective effects against hormone-associated cancers such as prostate cancer and breast cancer (*American Journal of Clinical Nutrition,* December 1995 supplement).

Q: **Have any studies looked at factors other than the link between vitamin C intake and cancer risk?**

A: Yes. Researchers have discovered that women with endometrial cancer, cervical cancer or cervical dysplasia (the presence of abnormal cells that may lead to cervical cancer) have lower levels of vitamin C in their blood than do women without those conditions.

One study, published in a 1988 issue of the *Journal of the National Cancer Institute,* found that these low plasma levels of vitamin C may increase the risk of cervical cancer. Women with the lowest blood levels of vitamin C were 60 percent more likely to have cervical cancer than were those with the highest blood levels.

Still other studies have linked cervical dysplasia with vitamin C deficiency. According to one study, women whose daily intake is less than half of the 60-milligram RDA are seven times more likely to develop cervical dysplasia than are women whose daily intake exceeds 60 milligrams.

Q: **That's interesting. Have any other links been found between vitamin C and cancer?**

A: Yes. Investigators have done some intriguing research relating to stomach cancer. British researchers in 1985 discovered that there may be a link between vitamin C levels in the stomach and the ability of stomach juices to promote potentially cancer-causing changes in cells in the stomach. The researchers found that the number of cell changes that can lead to stomach cancer were cut nearly in half after they gave study participants 4,000 milligrams (4 grams) of vitamin C a day for a week.

More recently, researchers obtained samples of stomach juices from 39 different people 30 and 60 minutes after injecting them with 500 milligrams of vitamin C and found that the levels of vitamin C in gastric juice varied based on a number of factors, including the patient's ethnic background, the pH level of the gastric juice (whether it was alkaline or acid) and the presence of *H. pylori,* a bacterium that has been implicated in stomach ulcers (*Journal of the National Cancer Institute,* January 4, 1995). This could mean that certain people might benefit from increasing their vitamin C intake.

Q: Anything else?

A: Yes. A study reported in the September 1996 *Epidemiology* examined the link between dietary intake of vitamin C and the risk of prostate cancer. While the researchers found no significant relationship between vitamin C intake and the development of prostate cancer, they did find that survival rates during the 30-year follow-up were higher in prostate cancer patients with high vitamin C intakes than in those with low vitamin C intakes.

Vitamin C and Cancer Treatment

Q: Have any studies specifically looked at vitamin C's ability to *treat* cancer?

A: Yes. But as we said at the beginning of this discussion, the results have not been conclusive. As a result, the use of vitamin C as a cancer treatment remains controversial.

Q: What started this controversy?

A: The controversy began in 1976, when Linus Pauling and Scottish surgeon Ewan Cameron published the results of a study in which they gave high doses of vitamin C— 10,000 milligrams (or 10 grams) per day—to 100 terminally ill cancer patients. Pauling and Cameron then compared the survival times of these patients with the survival times indicated in hospital records of 1,000 terminally ill cancer patients. They found that cancer patients who received high doses of vitamin C lived approximately 4.2 times longer than those who did not. Those given vitamin C lived an average of 210 days; those who did not receive vitamin C lived an average of 50 days (*Proceedings of the National Academy of Sciences,* October 1976).

Q: That sounds like pretty strong evidence. Where's the controversy?

A: The controversy lies in the research method Pauling and Cameron used, the failure of later studies to substantiate their findings and the research methods used by researchers in later studies.

Q: Let's take one thing at a time. What was the problem with Pauling and Cameron's research method?

A: The major complaint was that the control subjects— those who didn't receive vitamin C—didn't receive a placebo.

Q: Why is that important?

A: Researchers generally try to compare the effectiveness of the treatment they are testing with the effectiveness of an inactive, or placebo, treatment. This is done to rule out any effect that simply administering treatment might have on study participants.

Q: I don't understand. Could you explain further?

A: Many people feel better when they are given a treatment they think will work—regardless of whether that treatment actually has direct therapeutic value. This phenomenon is known as the placebo effect. To counter that effect, researchers generally give participants either the treatment or the placebo without telling them which they have received. Consequently, all of the participants believe that what they have been given may help them get better.

Q: I think I understand. You're saying that the people who received vitamin C in Pauling's study may have survived longer because they *believed* the vitamin C was helping them, right?

A: Right.

Q: So why didn't someone just repeat the study using a placebo?

A: Someone did. Researchers at the Mayo Clinic attempted to duplicate Pauling and Cameron's research, this time giving the control patients a placebo. They found no link between vitamin C and cancer survival.

Q: Didn't you say this later research was also controversial?

A: Yes. Pauling and others criticized the study because most of the participants—unlike those in the original study—had received chemotherapy or radiation treatments or both before they received the vitamin C. These treatments, they said, could have compromised the immune systems of the cancer patients to the point that they could not respond to vitamin C.

Q: What happened next?

A: The Mayo Clinic researchers conducted a second study. This study, reported in a 1985 issue of the *New England Journal of Medicine,* was limited to people with colon cancer that was not treated with chemotherapy. Again, researchers failed to find a link between vitamin C and cancer survival. And again, Pauling and others criticized the study.

Q: What was the criticism this time?

A: Primarily that the researchers did not allow adequate time to test Pauling's hypothesis. They withdrew the vitamin C treatment as soon as it became apparent that cancer had progressed. As a result, the participants in this study received vitamin C for only 2.5 months—a length of time Pauling said was too short to significantly extend the lives of people with terminal cancer.

Q: Was that the end of the story?

A: As far as the tit for tat, yes. While the Mayo studies did not substantiate Pauling and Cameron's findings that vitamin C can extend the survival time of people with terminal cancer, they did not refute them either.

Q: Have there been any studies since then?

A: Yes. Pauling and another colleague, Abram Hoffer, conducted a follow-up study in which they gave high amounts of vitamin C—12,000 milligrams (or 12 grams) per day—along with high doses of other nutrients to 101 cancer patients and compared the results with those of 31 cancer patients who did not receive supplements. Again, they found that high-dose vitamin C extended survival time (*Journal of Orthomolecular Medicine,* 1990).

Vitamin C's Cancer-Fighting Mechanisms

Q: **Have any researchers looked at** *how* **vitamin C might help cancer patients?**

A: Yes. Studies have shown that vitamin C can slow the growth of cancer cells and increase the cell-killing ability of cancer drugs.

Q: **That sounds promising. Could you give me an example or two?**

A: Certainly.

- In one recent study, researchers exposed two types of breast cancer cells to three anticancer drugs alone and in combination with vitamin C. In both types of cells, vitamin C showed an ability to destroy the cells (*Cancer Letters,* June 5, 1996).

- Researchers reported in a 1994 issue of *Nutrition and Cancer* that vitamin C was able to reduce the growth of melanoma (a deadly type of skin cancer) cells in test tubes.

Q: **Does vitamin C have any other possible benefits for cancer patients?**

A: Informal, unpublished accounts suggest that vitamin C may help reduce the side effects of radiation and chemotherapy treatments in cancer patients. And it is standard practice in many hospitals to give cancer patients vitamin C supplements.

Q: Why is that?

A: For two reasons: Many cancer patients have low blood levels of vitamin C and other nutrients, and vitamin C is essential for the proper functioning of the immune system.

Q: That reminds me. I know we discussed this briefly before, but how exactly is vitamin C thought to protect the body against cancer?

A: There are three primary methods. As we've just said, vitamin C is needed for the proper function of the immune system, which helps the body recognize and destroy abnormal, or precancerous, cells. In addition, vitamin C's antioxidant ability is thought to protect the genetic material of our cells (our DNA) from oxidative damage that can lead to cancer. Finally, vitamin C has been found to block the formation of **nitrosamines** and similar chemical compounds that increase the risk of cancer.

Q: I'm pretty clear on the first method, but I'd like more information about the other two. Have any studies actually looked at whether or not vitamin C can prevent damage to our cells' genetic material?

A: Yes, with contradictory results.

- In a recent study, researchers added vitamin C and vitamin E, both singly and together, to cells in test tubes, then exposed the cells to various doses of radiation or hydrogen peroxide in an effort to initiate an oxidative reaction. On examining the cells, the researchers found that the level of genetic damage to the cells supplemented with vitamin C was lower than the level of damage to the cells that weren't supplemented (*Nutrition and Cancer,* 1997).

• Researchers who gave 142 smokers vitamin C supplements in doses ranging from 250 to 500 milligrams found that the supplements did not affect the rate at which a substance that indicates oxidative genetic damage was eliminated from the body (*American Journal of Clinical Nutrition,* February 1997).

Q: **Is the evidence any better for vitamin C's ability to neutralize those substances you called nitrosamines?**

A: Yes. Several studies have shown that vitamin C can block the formation of nitrosamines. These substances are formed in the digestive tract from the nitrates and nitrites we ingest. (Nitrates and nitrites, often used as food preservatives, are found in cured packaged meats such as bacon, cold cuts and hot dogs.) By blocking the formation of these substances, vitamin C may be able to block the formation of tumors that the nitrosamines could generate, notably in the stomach.

Q: **I need a little bit of help putting this all in perspective. Could you tell me once again exactly how vitamin C may protect against cancer?**

A: Certainly. Studies indicate that vitamin C could provide a protective effect by:

• maintaining or improving the functioning of the immune system

- neutralizing free radicals, thus reducing the cellular damage that can lead to cancer

- slowing the growth of cancer cells

- increasing the cell-killing ability of cancer drugs

- blocking the formation of nitrosamines and similar compounds that increase the risk of cancer

Vitamin C and Colds

Q: OK, we've covered the "big C." What about the little c—the common cold? Does vitamin C really prevent it?

A: There is still disagreement in the health community about whether vitamin C actually prevents colds. While some studies support Linus Pauling's contention that it does, other studies indicate that it does not. However, many of these dissenting studies have found that vitamin C may decrease the length of colds and lessen the severity of cold symptoms.

Q: Could you tell me a little about these studies?

A: Certainly. Since 1970, when Pauling first recommended that people take vitamin C to prevent or fight colds, nearly 8,000 people have been given between 65 and 3,000 milligrams of vitamin C or a placebo every day for anywhere between eight weeks and nine months to determine if vitamin C has any effect on colds. In each of the studies, colds occurred.

A recent analysis of six studies in which vitamin C was given in doses of 1,000 milligrams (1 gram) or more did find, however, that supplements helped reduce the incidence of colds in certain groups of people. The analysis, reported in the January 1997 *British Medical Journal,* found that while vitamin C supplementation reduced the incidence of colds by only 1 percent—a result researchers consider insignificant—it reduced the incidence of colds in British male schoolchildren by 30 percent, leading the researchers to conclude that the vitamin can affect cold susceptibility in certain groups of people.

Q: **Have any other groups been identified?**

A: Yes. Studies indicate that people under heavy physical stress who take vitamin C are less susceptible to colds than those who don't take the vitamin.

Q: **What type of physical stress are you talking about?**

A: The studies looked at marathon runners, skiers and military recruits in training—in short, people who participate in intensive exercise.

Q: **What type of reduction in cold incidence do these people see?**

A: An analysis of three studies, reported in the July 1996 *International Journal of Sports Medicine,* found that doses between 600 and 1,000 milligrams per day of vitamin C reduced the incidence of colds by about 50 percent. Similar results were seen in a fourth study of skiers, but the study wasn't included in the analysis because none of the skiers received a placebo. A fifth study, however, saw no reduction in cold incidence in a group of military recruits.

Q: So the controversy of whether vitamin C reduces the number of colds people get still rages. But didn't you say that vitamin C may reduce the duration and severity of colds?

A: Yes. A number of studies have found that vitamin C reduces the duration and severity of colds. An analysis of 12 studies showed a 37 percent average reduction in the duration of colds treated with vitamin C in doses between 80 and 1,000 milligrams per day. And an analysis of 21 studies in which vitamin C was given in doses between 1,000 and 4,000 milligrams (1 and 4 grams) a day found a 23 percent reduction in cold duration. Many of the studies analyzed also found that cold symptoms were less severe in people who took vitamin C supplements.

Q: What do those percentages mean in terms of days? And which symptoms were less severe?

A: The percentages generally translate into a day or less, but the symptoms whose severity is decreased include such heavyweights as runny nose, watery eyes and cough.

Q: How does vitamin C fight colds?

A: There may be several ways. As we've said, white blood cells and other components of the immune system require vitamin C for normal functioning. And it is the immune system, after all, that protects us from the viruses that cause colds. Levels of vitamin C in the white blood cells drop during colds and other infections, implying that the vitamin plays a role in infection-fighting. And test-tube studies have shown that white blood cells treated with vitamin C fight more effectively against foreign invaders such as bacteria and viruses.

In addition, vitamin C stimulates the production of **interferon**, a protein excreted by cells that have been exposed to a virus. Interferon is thought to prevent the multiplication of the virus until other components of the immune system take over and destroy it.

Finally, vitamin C may reduce the severity of cold symptoms by lowering blood levels of **histamine**, a biochemical released by cells in the immune system that contributes to the runny noses of colds and allergies.

Q: Does vitamin C help fight any other type of respiratory infections?

A: It appears to. When British researchers gave 200 milligrams of vitamin C or a placebo to 57 elderly people hospitalized for bronchitis or pneumonia, those who got the vitamin C fared better than those who didn't (*International Journal of Vitamin and Nutrition Research,* July-September 1994). The researchers assessed the recovery of the study participants using a scoring system based on the major symptoms of respiratory infection. They theorized that vitamin C might have improved the immune response of the study participants. Or it might have protected them by neutralizing the free radicals generated by their immune system as they fought off the infections.

Fifty-five percent of the vitamin C produced in or imported to the United States is used in pharmaceutical preparations; 35 percent is used to fortify foods and beverages; and 10 percent is used in animal feed, according to Chemical Marketing Reporter *(January 1, 1996).*

VITAMIN C AND THE RESPIRATORY SYSTEM

Q: That reminds me: You mentioned back at the beginning of the chapter that vitamin C may help protect the lungs. How?

A: Vitamin C acts as an antioxidant in the lungs and, as such, may help protect lungs from the damaging effects of cigarette smoke and air pollutants. In general, it appears to improve lung function and may also help reduce asthma and allergy attacks.

Vitamin C and Smoking

Q: Didn't you say that smoking depletes the body of vitamin C?

A: We did. Numerous studies have found that smokers have lower levels of vitamin C in their blood and in their white blood cells than nonsmokers.

Q: Then how can vitamin C protect the lungs from cigarette smoke?

A: The theory is that the pollutants created by burning tobacco contribute to the production of free radicals, which, as you know, have been implicated in a variety of conditions including cancer, heart disease and other diseases for which smokers are at risk. Vitamin C, an antioxidant, neutralizes these harmful free radicals and, in the process, blood levels of it are depleted. (As you may recall, when an antioxidant neutralizes a free radical, it becomes inactive.) The more smoke a person breathes, the more free radicals are produced and the more vitamin C is used up fighting them. This is why the RDA for smokers is nearly twice that for nonsmokers.

Q: **What about nonsmokers who breathe in cigarette smoke? They're exposed to the same pollutants, although in smaller quantities. Do they need more vitamin C than people who don't breathe in secondhand smoke?**

A: It appears so. Researchers at the Stanford Center for Research in Disease Prevention reported in 1993 that nonsmokers exposed to cigarette smoke for more than 20 hours a week have lower blood levels of vitamin C than nonsmokers who aren't exposed to smoke—even if their vitamin C intakes are the same.

Q: **But these lower levels mean that vitamin C is protecting the lungs, right?**

A: Right, although this protection can result in vitamin C deficiencies. Fortunately, studies show that these blood levels of vitamin C increase when vitamin C intake increases.

Q: **Does exposure to other air pollutants also deplete vitamin C?**

A: Yes. In studies, exposure to air pollutants such as ozone depletes vitamin C in the lungs, which implies that the vitamin is exerting a protective effect.

Vitamin C and Lung Function

Q: Didn't you say there's evidence that vitamin C can actually improve lung function?

A: Yes. Several studies have found that vitamin C intake increases performance on **pulmonary function tests**—tests that determine how well the lungs are performing.

- In one study, reported in the January 1994 *American Journal of Clinical Nutrition,* adults with high intakes of vitamin C performed better on the forced expiratory volume test (a test that measures the greatest amount of air that can be expelled in one second when a person exhales as hard as possible) than did adults with low intakes of vitamin C.

- Cambridge University researchers reported in the September 1996 *European Journal of Clinical Nutrition* that men with high plasma levels of vitamin C performed better on two pulmonary function tests—forced expiratory volume and forced vital capacity, a test that measures the total amount of air that can be exhaled as rapidly as possible—than did men with low plasma levels. The association between vitamin C levels and test performance was weaker for women, however.

- A study reported in the May 1995 *American Journal of Respiratory and Critical Care Medicine* looked at the diets and lung function of 2,633 people and found that the difference in lung function between those who took in the most vitamin C and those who took in the least was comparable to the difference between people who smoke a pack of cigarettes a day for five to seven years and nonsmokers. The benefit came from an average daily intake of 99 milligrams.

Vitamin C and Asthma

Q: What effect does vitamin C have on asthma?

A: Asthma, a respiratory disease in which air passages in the lungs periodically become narrowed or obstructed, can be triggered by tobacco smoke and other air pollutants. As we've said, vitamin C may reduce the harmful effects of smoke and other pollutants and improve lung function and, so, reduce asthma's effects. But there may be more to it than that.

Q: Such as?

A: Some research shows that the risk of asthma and other respiratory disease goes down as vitamin C intake goes up (*Tufts University Diet and Nutrition Letter,* February 1996).

Q: Wait a minute. Do you mean that vitamin C intake can actually decrease the risk of asthma?

A: Possibly. A review article published in a March 1995 supplement to the *American Journal of Clinical Nutrition* notes that vitamin C intake in the general population appears to correlate with asthma, suggesting that a diet low in vitamin C is a risk factor for asthma.

Q: What other possible connections have been uncovered between vitamin C and asthma?

A: Studies show that blood and white blood cell concentrations of vitamin C are lower in people with asthma than in people without asthma. And more than half a dozen studies show improved breathing in people with asthma who receive vitamin C supplements.

The most recent study, reported in the April 1997 *Archives of Pediatrics and Adolescent Medicine,* found that vitamin C may help prevent or reduce the severity of asthma symptoms in young people whose asthma is triggered by exercise. The researchers gave 20 youngsters either 2,000 milligrams (2 grams) of vitamin C or a placebo before asking them to perform a seven-minute exercise session on a treadmill. The vitamin C supplements prevented asthma symptoms in nine of the youngsters and reduced the severity of symptoms in two others.

Q: I can understand how vitamin C may counter asthma triggered by pollutants or smoke, but exercise? What's the connection?

A: It's not actually a connection to exercise, but rather a connection to the disease itself. During an asthma attack, the linings of the bronchial tubes become inflamed and swollen. This inflammation is thought to be caused by an overactive immune system. As you may recall, the immune system deliberately makes free radicals to destroy bacteria, viruses and other harmful organisms. The researchers speculate that these free radicals may contribute to asthma and that vitamin C may neutralize them.

Q: Can't asthma also be triggered by allergies?

A: Yes, it can.

Q: And you said vitamin C may also reduce allergy attacks, right?

A: Right. As we've said, vitamin C has been shown to lower blood levels of histamine, the immune system mediator, or chemical, that triggers tissue inflammation, runny noses and watery eyes.

VITAMIN C AND THE EYES

Q: Speaking of eyes, how is vitamin C thought to protect against cataracts?

A: Cataracts, the clouding of the eye's transparent lens, are thought to occur when proteins in the eye become oxidized, often as a result of sun exposure. Vitamin C is thought to protect the eye against this oxidative damage.

Q: Is there any evidence that it does this?

A: Yes. Test-tube and animal studies support this hypothesis, and several epidemiological studies indicate that it may hold true in people as well. At least five studies have shown that people with high blood levels of vitamin C have a reduced risk of cataracts, and three studies have shown that people who take multivitamin supplements, which include vitamin C, have a reduced risk.

Still, the research is not conclusive. In one study, Chinese adults given 120 milligrams of vitamin C a day for five years had no fewer cataracts than counterparts who took a placebo. And while women in the Nurses' Health Study who took vitamin C supplements for 10 or more years were 45 percent less likely to have cataract surgery than women who did not take supplements, men who took vitamin C and E supplements for six years as part of the Physicians' Health Study saw no reduction in cataract risk.

Q: **Could the different lengths of the studies have any effect on the results?**

A: Possibly. Tufts University researchers who conducted a follow-up study on 247 Boston-area women who participated in the nurses' study found that those who used vitamin C supplements for 10 or more years had a 77 percent lower incidence of early lens clouding—the first sign of cataracts—than women who did not take vitamin C supplements. But women who took vitamin C supplements for fewer than 10 years had no reduction in incidence of lens clouding (*American Journal of Clinical Nutrition,* October 1997). The researchers concluded that long-term supplementation may be necessary to reduce the risk of cataract development.

Q: **Does vitamin C have any other effects on the eye?**

A: Possibly. Vitamin C concentrations in the lens of the eye are up to 60 times higher than those in the blood, which implies that the vitamin does indeed play a role in eye health.

It may, for example, help protect against age-related **macular degeneration,** a breakdown of the **macula** that is the leading cause of irreversible blindness among older adults. Research conducted by investigators at Harvard Medical School and several leading eye institutes found a significantly lower risk of macular degeneration in people who ate a diet rich in dark green leafy and yellow or red vegetables and other foods high in antioxidant vitamins. While the largest benefit was seen in foods containing high amounts of the **carotenoids** lutein and zeaxanthin—the dominant pigments in the macula—foods high in vitamin C also conferred some benefit (*Journal of the American Medical Association,* November 9, 1994).

Q: Anything else?

A: Vitamin C and other antioxidant nutrients may also play a role in slowing the progression of macular degeneration. In an 18-month study of older U.S. veterans with advanced macular degeneration, those who took an over-the-counter supplement that contained 750 milligrams of vitamin C, along with vitamin E, beta carotene, selenium and other nutrients, saw their vision stabilize, while those who took a placebo saw their vision deteriorate (*Journal of the American Optometric Association,* January 1996).

VITAMIN C AND THE SKIN

Q: What is vitamin C's connection to the skin?

A: As you may recall, vitamin C is essential for the production of collagen, the protein that helps support and maintain the structure of the skin and other tissues.

Collagen helps skin look smooth, gives it resilience and lessens the likelihood of wrinkles.

Q: **Does vitamin C actually protect the skin in any way?**

A: It appears to. There is evidence that vitamin C may help heal burns, speed wound healing and reduce scar formation.

Q: **How is it thought to do these things?**

A: In all three cases, vitamin C's essential roles in immune function and collagen production combine to reduce the risk of infection and stimulate tissue repair.

Q: **What do studies show?**

A: It is well documented that vitamin C deficiencies lead to slower wound healing. And a study by British researchers of people confined to bed because of hip fractures found that low white blood cell levels of vitamin C increased the risk of developing pressure sores, or bedsores.

Higher blood levels of vitamin C, on the other hand, appear to offer a protective effect. For example, a 1982 review of studies of patients recovering from surgery, injuries, pressure sores and leg ulcers found that vitamin C supplements in doses ranging from 500 to 3,000 milligrams can speed wound healing in people who are not vitamin-C deficient. Other studies have found that vitamin C can speed the healing of burns or lessen their severity and reduce scar formation.

Q: **Does vitamin C have any other effects on the skin?**

A: There is some evidence that topical vitamin C may protect the skin from ultraviolet light, which damages the skin and can lead to skin cancer.

In studies reviewed at a 1996 meeting of the Gerontological Society of America, researchers reported that the skins of live pigs were protected from sunburn and cellular damage when they were treated with topical vitamin C, then exposed to ultraviolet light.

And researcher Sheldon Pinnell, chief of dermatology at Duke University Medical Center in Durham, North Carolina, reported at a 1996 American Academy of Dermatology news briefing that a form of topical vitamin C sold under the brand name Cellex-C may help reduce wrinkling and other sun damage in humans. Five volunteers who used the compound every day for eight months saw reductions in wrinkling on the half of their face that received the compound. Pinnell theorized that the vitamin compound may soak up free radicals created by sun exposure.

OTHER VITAMIN C USES

Q: **At the beginning of the chapter, you mentioned several other conditions for which vitamin C may be of benefit, but I can't remember what they are. Could you refresh my memory?**

A: Certainly. In recent years, researchers have found several connections between vitamin C and **diabetes**

and between vitamin C and osteoarthritis. Reports have also linked the vitamin to improved mental health, increased fertility and improved bone density and muscle recovery.

Vitamin C and Diabetes

Q: Let's start with diabetes. What exactly is it?

A: Diabetes is a disease resulting from the body's inability to produce or use **insulin**, a hormone that enables the body to use sugar for energy. The disease is characterized by an abnormally high concentration of sugar in the bloodstream.

Q: What links have researchers found between it and vitamin C?

A: Levels of vitamin C in the blood and in the white blood cells are often low in people with diabetes, making them susceptible to gum disease, slow wound healing and rapidly aging skin as well as high cholesterol levels and atherosclerosis.

People with diabetes are also more likely to suffer from complications from atherosclerosis than other people. Research indicates that this increased risk may stem from low levels of insulin, which have been shown in test-tube studies to reduce the amount of vitamin C taken in by cells.

Q: Can these problems be alleviated by increasing vitamin C intake?

A: Some can. Animal studies indicate that vitamin C supplements may help diabetic people overcome gum disease, slow wound healing and rapidly aging skin. And new research indicates that vitamin C may help reduce several other diabetic complications, including circulatory problems that can lead to eye and kidney problems, among other things.

Q: What's the connection between vitamin C and circulation?

A: Harvard University researchers have found that vitamin C can increase circulation in people with non-insulin-dependent diabetes by helping their blood vessels dilate. Researchers gave diabetic people a vessel-dilating drug— either alone or with injections of vitamin C—and found that those given the vitamin C experienced a 36 percent increase in blood flow compared with those who received the drug alone (*Journal of Clinical Investigation,* January 1996).

Q: That sounds like those studies of smokers and people with coronary-artery disease you mentioned earlier.

A: Yes. As you recall, German researchers found that the blood vessels of smokers and people with coronary-artery disease opened up more when they were given vitamin C along with a vessel-dilating drug than when they were given the drug alone.

They theorized that the vitamin was able to counter damage to the endothelium, the cells lining the blood vessel walls.

Q: Does the same theory hold for the diabetes study?

A: Yes. Experts have long associated the impaired vascular function of people with diabetes to endo-thelial damage. The Harvard researchers believe that vitamin C improved the performance of the endothelial cells. The re-searchers believe that this finding supports the theory that free radicals cause blood vessels to react abnormally in people with diabetes. They note that high blood sugar causes proteins to link at a higher rate, which may trigger the production of excess free radicals in people with diabetes.

Q: Didn't you say that improving blood vessel function might help reduce the risk of other diabetic complications?

A: Yes. It might help prevent several complications that are linked to poor blood vessel function—notably **retinopathy** (a disease of the blood vessels in the retina of the eye), **nephropathy** (kidney disease) and atherosclerosis.

Q: Is there any other way that vitamin C might benefit people with diabetes?

A: Yes. Vitamin C may stop the body from producing **sorbitol**, a sugar alcohol that may contribute to kid-ney, retina and nerve damage. In a recent study, researchers gave either 100 or 600 milligrams of vitamin C to nine people with diabetes and 11 people without diabetes. Diabetic people who had higher than average levels of sorbitol at the start of the study saw a reduction in sorbitol levels; levels remained the same in people without diabetes (*Journal of the American College of Nutrition,* August 1994).

Vitamin C and Osteoarthritis

Q: What's the connection between vitamin C and osteoarthritis?

A: An important study published in the April 1996 *Arthritis and Rheumatism* found that a high dietary intake of antioxidant nutrients, particularly vitamin C, may slow the progression of osteoarthritis, or "wear-and-tear" arthritis.

Researchers at Boston University Medical Center analyzed information collected from 640 people who participated in the Framingham Osteoarthritis Cohort Study and found that a moderate to high intake of vitamin C (150 to 400 milligrams per day) protected against the progression of osteoarthritis of the knee. Specifically, the study found that people whose diets included at least 150 milligrams of vitamin C were three times less likely to have their arthritis progress during the 10-year study period than were those whose diets were lower in vitamin C. Those who took in 400 milligrams a day experienced a similar slowing and were also less likely to experience knee pain.

A report in the July 1997 *Annals of the Rheumatic Diseases* lends credence to these findings, citing the Framingham study and several others that have found a connection between antioxidants and improvement of osteoarthritis.

Vitamin C and Mental Health

Q: How is vitamin C related to mental health?

A: At least one study indicates that people with psychiatric problems have lower plasma levels of vitamin C than healthy individuals.

Q: Does vitamin C show any promise as a treatment for mental disorders?

A: Yes. Research indicates that it may be useful in the treatment of mental disorders such as **schizophrenia**, which is characterized by an abnormal perception and thought process, and **manic depression**, or **bipolar disorder**, which is characterized by alternating bouts of depression and energetic, impulsive behavior.

Q: In what way might vitamin C be useful in treating these conditions?

A: Either alone or in combination with drugs. In one small study, high doses of vitamin C—8,000 milligrams (8 grams) per day—were found to improve depressive, manic and paranoid symptoms in 10 out of 13 patients with schizophrenia. High doses of vitamin C have also been used successfully to treat manic depression in two small studies.

And vitamin C has been found to enhance the effectiveness of haloperidol, a drug widely used to treat severe mental illness, which may make it possible to reduce dosages of the drug and, so, reduce its side effects.

Q: Does vitamin C have any other effects on mental health?

A: One study indicates that it may improve cognitive function—such things as memory, logic, perception and orientation—in elderly individuals. Researchers followed 921 randomly selected seniors for 20 years and found that cognitive function was poorest in those with the lowest blood levels or intake of vitamin C (*British Medical Journal,* March 9, 1996). The researchers noted that while a low vitamin C status could simply be a consequence of cognitive impairment, it could also be a cause.

Q: In what way?

A: The researchers believe that vitamin C might protect against declining cognitive function through its antioxidant activity and its ability to help prevent or slow the progression of atherosclerosis, which can affect blood vessels in the brain.

Vitamin C and Infertility

Q: What link does vitamin C have to infertility?

A: It may actually have several links—at least to male infertility.

The concentration of vitamin C is higher in the testicles than in the blood, but many men with infertility problems have low testicular levels of vitamin C.

Studies have also shown that men with low intakes of vitamin C have increased levels in their sperm of a substance that indicates oxidative damage to the genetic material in cells. So vitamin C clearly has some connection to male fertility.

Q: Can vitamin C actually combat male infertility problems?

A: It appears so, in some cases.

Researchers have found that a common form of male infertility, caused by sperm cells clumping together, can be reversed with daily supplements of about 1,000 milligrams (1 gram) of vitamin C. The supplements increased sperm count and sperm function and improved sperm motility (movement).

Vitamin C and Bones

Q: What effect does vitamin C have on bones?

A: Researchers from the Loma Linda University School of Medicine and the University of California, Los Angeles, School of Medicine reported in 1996 that dietary vitamin C may increase the bone mineral density of post-menopausal women.

The researchers compared the dietary histories and bone mineral densities of 775 postmenopausal women and found that those who ate a diet rich in vitamin C had higher femoral, neck and total hip bone mineral densities than women who ate few vitamin-C rich foods. The researchers found that every additional 100 milligrams of vitamin C a woman consumed per day corresponded with a 2 to 2.5 percent increase in total bone mineral density.

Vitamin C and Muscles

Q: What effect does vitamin C have on muscle recovery?

A: A small study reported in the *European Journal of Applied Physiology* in 1993 found that people who took 400 milligrams of vitamin C had greater recovery of muscle strength after a 60-minute rigorous workout than did those who took 400 milligrams of vitamin E or those who took a placebo. Those who took the vitamin C also reported less muscle soreness in the 24 hours after the workout. Study participants took the supplements for three weeks before and one week after the workout, and muscle strength was measured before and after.

Q: To what did the researchers attribute the recovery?

A: They theorized that vitamin C neutralized the free radicals released by exercise.

PUTTING IT ALL TOGETHER

Q: Now that we've gone through all the research, I'm still somewhat confused. Some of the research seems to indicate that vitamin C has some real health benefits, but some of it doesn't. Why the discrepancy?

A: There are a number of possible reasons. One of the primary ones involves the research itself. Investigators use a variety of research techniques, and these various techniques often create differing results. This is perfectly normal—in fact, these differing results are necessary to test theories and build consensus among research findings.

Q: In what way?

A: Let's look at the apparently conflicting research on vitamin C and cancer, for example. This research, like research on many other subjects, began with epidemiological studies—studies designed to find the possible link between a disease or condition and its causes or preventives.

In this instance, researchers were attempting to determine if there was a link between diet and cancer. They compared the diets of various groups of people with their risk of developing cancer and, in nearly all cases, found that people who eat the most fruits and vegetables are less likely to develop cancer than those who eat the least. Researchers then theorized that fruits or vegetables—or some component or components in them—protect against cancer.

Q: That certainly sounds like a reasonable conclusion. What's the problem?

A: There is no problem. But the studies don't actually indicate that vitamin C offers cancer protection; they simply indicate that fruits and vegetables—or some component thereof—have a protective effect. To find out if that component is vitamin C, more research is needed.

Q: What kind of research?

A: Research that isolates the effects of vitamin C from the effects of other components in fruits and vegetables.

Q: Are you talking about research into vitamin C supplements?

A: Yes. And research into blood levels of vitamin C, and research into vitamin C's actions on cancer cells and so on—any areas of research that look specifically at the link between vitamin C and cancer.

Q: Aren't these the type of studies that have provided conflicting results?

A: Yes. These studies examine a wide variety of issues using a wide variety of research methods. Because they differ in both subject matter and method, they often produce differing results.

Q: But how can you explain the discrepancy between these results and the findings of the studies that link diets high in fruits and vegetables to cancer prevention? Those studies all seemed to reach the same conclusions.

A: They did and, in fact, it's now fairly well accepted that a diet rich in fruit and vegetables—and, consequently, rich in vitamin C—can help protect against cancer. The apparently conflicting studies do not disprove this; they simply fail to link vitamin C directly to this protective effect. It could be that other nutrients in fruits and vegetables are responsible for the protective effect or that vitamin C offers protection only when it works in combination with other nutrients. Or it could be that vitamin C offers protection only against certain types of cancer or only to certain people. These are the very issues further research will ultimately help determine.

Each study reveals a new piece of the puzzle. When enough pieces become available, we will have our solution. Until that time, however, we simply don't have all the answers. This holds for other areas of vitamin C research as well.

Q: But what should we do in the meantime?

A: Be aware of the research findings to date and keep track of new findings as they emerge. You may have already drawn some conclusions about vitamin C's various health benefits, or you may need more information before you can do so. And your conclusion, like the research findings themselves, may change in the future.

3 WHAT ELSE DO I NEED TO KNOW?

Q: Even if only a few of the claims made for vitamin C are ultimately substantiated, am I right in assuming that the vitamin is pretty important to our health and well-being?

A: Yes. In fact, it's already been proven that vitamin C is necessary for the body to function normally—that's why it's been labeled a vitamin.

DOSAGE

Q: How much vitamin C do we need to stay healthy and prevent disease?

A: You're asking two different questions. As you may recall from the preceding chapters, the amounts recommended to stay healthy—in other words, to prevent deficiency symptoms—are generally not the same as the amounts that have been linked to disease prevention.

Q: OK. Let's address them one at a time. How much vitamin C do we need to stay healthy?

A: As we said in chapter 1, the Recommended Dietary Allowance (RDA) for vitamin C is 60 milligrams per day for adult men and women and 100 milligrams per day for smokers. RDAs for other groups range from 30 milligrams per day for infants up to six months old to 95 milligrams per day for breast-feeding women in their first six months of lactation. The chart that follows gives the daily RDAs for all gender and age-groups.

Recommended Dietary Allowances for Vitamin C

Category	Age	Amount in milligrams
Infants	0-6 months	30
	6 months-1 year	35
Children	1-3 years	40
	4-10 years	45
	11-14 years	50
Men	15+ years	60
Women	15+ years	60
	Pregnant	70
	Lactating (1st 6 months)	95
	Lactating (2nd 6 months)	90
Smokers		100

Q: Refresh my memory. What exactly do these recommendations mean?

A: The RDAs are levels of nutrient intake—from either foods or supplements—that the National Academy of Sciences' Food and Nutrition Board believes to be adequate to meet the known nutrient needs of practically all healthy people.

These amounts go somewhat beyond what is needed to prevent deficiency-related diseases—in fact, it's possible to consistently take in less than the RDA for a particular nutrient and not suffer adverse

Studies show that at least 20 to 30 percent of American adults take in less than the 60-milligram RDA.

health problems as a result. The amount of vitamin C needed to prevent scurvy, for example, is 10 milligrams—well below the 60-milligram RDA. On the other hand, amounts higher than the RDA may be necessary for optimal health.

Q: Before we go on, could you tell me again what the symptoms of scurvy and vitamin C deficiency are?

A: Certainly. Symptoms of mild deficiencies include easy bruising, delayed wound healing and reduced resistance to infections. Serious deficiencies can result in scurvy, which is characterized by bleeding gums, loose teeth, joint tenderness and swelling, extreme weakness and fatigue, hemorrhaging under the skin, anemia and poor wound healing.

Q: And the RDAs are designed to prevent these symptoms. But didn't you say in chapter 1 that the RDAs are undergoing review?

A: Yes. The Food and Nutrition Board is in the process of revising the RDAs so that they will take into consideration not only the amount of each nutrient that is needed to prevent deficiency diseases but also the amount needed to decrease the risk of chronic diseases such as cancer and heart disease. These revised RDAs will become part of a new set of figures known as Dietary Reference Intakes (DRIs).

Q: When will the DRIs for vitamin C be available?

A: The Food and Nutrition Board hopes to establish DRIs for all essential nutrients by the year 2000, but it has not established a precise time frame for the release of the new recommendations.

Q: In the meantime, how do we know how much vitamin C we need to reduce our risk of chronic diseases and reap the vitamin's full benefits?

A: The answer depends on whom you ask. Vitamin C proponents such as the late Linus Pauling have recommended high doses of vitamin C—doses of 1,000 milligrams (1 gram) or more—to maintain health and help fight illnesses; those who are more skeptical of vitamin C's abilities, those who believe that amounts above a certain level offer no additional benefit and those who fear potential side effects from large doses generally recommend doses closer to the RDA; still others recommend levels somewhere in between.

Q: Why such a discrepancy?

A: For two primary reasons: The one universal recommendation we have—the RDA—does not address this optimal amount; and studies on vitamin C's protective effects cover a wide range of dosages. Some studies indicate that vitamin C confers health benefits at levels only slightly above the RDA; others have found benefits only at much higher levels.

Q: Has anyone attempted to put all this information together to come up with a scientifically valid recommendation?

A: Yes. In an article published in the December 1995 supplement to the *American Journal of Clinical Nutrition,* researchers from the National Institutes of Health outlined the criteria they believe must be used to determine an optimal intake of vitamin C.

Specifically, they believe that the intake should be based upon the relationship between the dose of the vitamin and its functions in the body, availability in the food supply, the amount needed to maintain steady levels of vitamin C in plasma and tissues, the level at which excess is eliminated in the urine, toxicity, epidemiologic observations and **bioavailability** (the degree to which a nutrient becomes available for use in the body after it has been ingested). Unfortunately, not all of this information is available.

Q: So what did they determine?

A: Based on the information available at the time, they determined that optimal vitamin C intake is anywhere between 6 and 750 milligrams.

Q: That's quite a range! Were they able to make any recommendations based on their research?

A: Yes. They suggested that people should try to get about 200 milligrams of vitamin C daily—an amount that can generally be obtained from five servings of fruit and vegetables. In fact, they suggested that people try to get their vitamin C from foods. And they said daily intake should not exceed 500 milligrams.

Q: Why not?

A: Because studies show that at doses above that level, the body tends to eliminate more **oxalate** in the urine. This salt, a product of vitamin C metabolism, has been linked to kidney stones. We discuss this link later in the chapter.

Q: OK. Has any information become available since they made their recommendations?

A: Yes. The same researchers reported in 1996 that doses of 200 milligrams a day appeared to be optimal and recommended that the RDA be increased to that level.

The following fruits provide 50 percent or more of the RDA for vitamin C in a single 3½ ounce serving: breadfruit, cantaloupe, currants, grapefruit, guava, honeydew, kiwifruit, lemon, orange, papaya, passion fruit, persimmons, strawberries and watermelon.

Q: How did they come to this conclusion?

A: It was the result of several studies—test-tube studies that examined vitamin C transport throughout the body and its function in white blood cells and a clinical study of seven healthy men.

Q: What was the study of the men about?

A: That study, reported in the April 16, 1996, *Proceedings of the National Academy of Sciences,* looked at the effects that varying dosages of vitamin C had on their plasma vitamin C levels. The men were hospitalized for four to six months and given a vitamin C-free diet. When their plasma vitamin C levels decreased as far as they could, the men were given daily doses of the vitamin ranging from 30 to 2,500 milligrams. At each dose, researchers calculated plasma concentrations, bioavailability, urinary elimination, toxicity and vitamin concentration in at least three different cells or tissues.

Q: What did they find?

A: They found that the blood becomes almost fully saturated with vitamin C at doses of 200 milligrams.

Bioavailability, too, peaks at doses of 200 milligrams. In higher doses, bioavailability levels dropped, and the amount of vitamin C eliminated in the urine increased. (Remember: Vitamin C is water soluble; amounts that aren't used by the body are eliminated in the urine.) These results led them to conclude that 200 milligrams is the ideal daily intake.

Q: **That seems to be pretty definitive, right?**

A: The findings are the most definitive yet in terms of vitamin C absorption, and the Food and Nutrition Board will likely take them into consideration when it develops the DRIs for vitamin C. But a number of questions still remain unanswered.

Q: **Such as?**

A: Such as how much vitamin C we need to optimize the functioning of our immune system, how much vitamin C we need to prevent degenerative diseases, how much vitamin C is needed by smokers and other populations and how much vitamin C we need when we are ill. Remember: The study that prompted the 200-milligram recommendation was a study of healthy men.

Q: **So I guess more research is needed, right?**

A: Right. As you may recall from the previous chapters, stress, illness, smoking and exposure to other environmental pollutants deplete the body of vitamin C. Thus, actual needs and optimal intakes may vary from individual to individual, from situation to situation and even, in some cases, from day to day. For example, you may need more vitamin C than you normally do when you're fighting a cold or infection or when you're exposed to tobacco smoke. Women typically need more vitamin C when they are pregnant or lactating (thus, the higher RDAs). And preliminary research indicates that pregnant women who smoke may need to take in twice as much vitamin C as pregnant women who don't smoke.

Q: Why is that?

A: Because pregnant smokers—and their fetuses—tend to have lower concentrations of vitamin C in their blood. Researchers from Our Lady of Mercy Medical Center in New York reported in 1995 that while newborns typically have twice the vitamin C concentrations of their mothers, newborns of smokers they studied had only 1.5 times the amount of vitamin C as their mothers.

TOXICITY

Q: Does anyone need **megadoses** of vitamin C?

A: That depends on what you mean by the word megadose. Some people use the word to define large doses or doses that exceed recommendations. In scientific terms, it has been defined as a dose that is 10 times the RDA or more. In the case of vitamin C, this would be a dose that is 600 milligrams or more—rather small in comparison with the high doses advocated by some people.

Q: OK. I'll reword my question. Does anybody need the multiple-gram doses that some people recommend?

A: There's not enough information available to make that determination, but just as high doses of vitamin C have been recommended by some people, they've been cautioned against by others.

Q: Why? I thought you said vitamin C is considered relatively safe even in large amounts.

A: It is. Excess amounts of vitamin C are generally eliminated in urine, which, incidentally, is one of the most commonly heard arguments against high doses: that the vitamin—and the money spent on it—literally goes down the drain. But high doses of vitamin C are known to cause abdominal cramping and diarrhea in some people; they have also been linked to kidney stones.

Q: I want to know more about that link, but first I want more details on the gastrointestinal side effects. At what dosage do they occur?

A: The dosage at which these symptoms occur, known as **bowel intolerance**, varies from person to person. Some people experience these effects from doses as low as 500 milligrams, but the symptoms generally do not occur until doses exceed several grams (1 gram is equal to 1,000 milligrams).

Q: **Are these symptoms dangerous?**

A: No. In fact, some proponents of high-dose supplementation use bowel intolerance as a guide to determine how much vitamin C a particular person needs. They recommend that a person take increasing amounts of vitamin C until symptoms appear, then cut back till they disappear: The level at which the symptoms disappear is considered to be optimal for that person.

Q: **So the symptoms just go away when the intake goes down?**

A: Yes.

Q: **That's reassuring. But what about the link between vitamin C and kidney stones?**

A: This side effect, while obviously more serious than the gastrointestinal problems we just discussed, is, fortunately, less common. In fact, it's rather controversial.

Even though there have been reports over the years that vitamin C increases the risk of developing kidney stones, no studies to date have shown a relationship between vitamin C and the formation of kidney stones in healthy people.

In fact, Harvard University researchers found no association between vitamin C intake and kidney stones in a recent study. Men who consumed the most vitamin C—1,500 milligrams (1.5 grams) or more per day—were at no greater risk of developing stones than men who consumed less than 250 milligrams.

Q: Then why has the vitamin been linked to kidney stones?

A: Primarily because when the body metabolizes, or breaks down, vitamin C, it produces **oxalic acid**, a common component in kidney stones. Indeed, the National Institutes of Health researchers who recommended that the RDA of vitamin C be increased to 200 milligrams found that the men eliminated more oxalate (an oxalic acid salt) in their urine when they took in 1,000 milligrams (1 gram) of vitamin C a day. They also eliminated more **urate**, a salt of **uric acid**. Uric acid, a crystalline substance found in urine, is also associated with stone formation and with **gout**, a type of arthritis. These findings underscore recommendations that people who are prone to kidney stones or who have kidney disease or gout should not use vitamin C supplements without the advice of their physicians.

Q: Why did you include kidney disease in that list?

A: Because the kidneys play an important role in ridding the body of excess vitamin C. If they aren't functioning properly, the body may not be able to get rid of excess vitamin C.

Q: Do excessive doses have any other side effects?

A: There have been reports that when high doses of vitamin C are discontinued suddenly, "rebound scurvy" may develop, but a recent review found that this is not the case. Still, experts advise that you reduce your intake gradually if you have been taking high doses of vitamin C.

Q: Anything else?

A: An article published in the June 1996 *Journal of Nutrition* raises the possibility that high doses of vitamin C, in the presence of high levels of iron in the body, may actually promote oxidation, generating harmful free radicals.

Q: How can vitamin C promote oxidation? It's an antioxidant.

A: As you may recall from chapter 1, oxidation occurs when unstable molecules or atoms known as free radicals steal electrons from other molecules or atoms. Antioxidants, such as vitamin C, donate electrons to these free radicals, thus stopping their thieving behavior. In the process, the antioxidants themselves become unbalanced. Generally, this simply renders them inactive. But in certain situations, this lack of balance can cause them to promote oxidation, or become **pro-oxidant**.

Q: That doesn't sound good. Is there a lot of evidence that vitamin C can do this?

A: The evidence to date is based on laboratory findings. No large studies have proven that vitamin C has a harmful, pro-oxidant effect on people's health.

Q: Are there any reasons for caution?

A: High doses of vitamin C may interfere with certain medical tests, notably tests to determine if there is hidden blood in the stool, such as the fecal occult blood test; tests to monitor blood sugar levels in people with diabetes; and tests to determine how much oxalate is in the urine, which are used to help diagnose kidney problems. Any time you undergo these and other laboratory tests, make sure to tell your practitioner and the laboratory technician what vitamins, minerals, other supplements and drugs you are taking.

DRUG INTERACTIONS

Q: **Speaking of drugs, does vitamin C interact with any?**

A: Yes. Both animal and human studies indicate that aspirin may block the absorption of vitamin C. Plasma, white blood cell and urinary levels of vitamin C are considerably lower and absorption rates are delayed when aspirin and vitamin C are given together, which could mean that people who use aspirin on a regular basis may need more vitamin C.

Q: **Have any other interactions been identified?**

A: Yes, although not all have been substantiated or proven to be significant. According to Joe and Teresa Graedon, authors of *The People's Guide to Deadly Drug Interactions,* vitamin C in doses of 1,000 milligrams (1 gram) or more may increase blood levels of estrogen, making side effects of oral contraceptives more noticeable. In doses of 5,000 milligrams (5 grams) or more, vitamin C may interfere with the effectiveness of blood-thinning drugs such as warfarin (Coumadin).

And large doses of vitamin C have also been reported to reduce blood levels of the tranquilizer fluphenazine (Prolixin).

In addition, the Graedons note that, like aspirin, other drugs may interfere with vitamin C absorption. These include alcohol and drugs in the tetracycline family of antibiotics, which includes Sumycin, Achromycin and Panmycin.

NUTRIENT INTERACTIONS

Q: **What about other nutrients? Does vitamin C interact with them in any way?**

A: Yes. But not all of vitamin C's interactions with other nutrients are harmful. As we said in chapter 1, vitamin C plays a role in the metabolism and utilization of folic acid and iron: It plays a role in converting folic acid, a B vitamin, into its biologically active form, and it helps our bodies absorb and use iron.

Q: But can't we get too much iron?

A: Yes. While vitamin C's role in increasing iron absorption may be a blessing for people who don't get enough iron, it can be a problem for people with hemochromatosis, a hereditary disorder in which too much iron builds up in the body. People who have this condition should monitor their vitamin C intake accordingly.

Still, recent research indicates that vitamin C may not play as great a role in iron absorption and use as was once thought. Researchers studied the effects of vitamin C supplementation, in doses of 1,500 milligrams (1.5 grams) a day, on women with low iron stores and found that while the vitamin slightly increased blood levels of ferritin (a form of iron), it did not affect half-life, iron absorption rates or several other biochemical measurements of iron status (*Journal of Clinical Nutrition,* June 1994). In other words, while it did have some effect on the body's use of iron, the effect was minimal.

Q: Didn't you say that vitamin C is also linked to vitamin E?

A: Yes. Several studies indicate that vitamin C may donate electrons to vitamin E after it has donated its own electrons to free radicals in an attempt to neutralize an oxidative reaction.

As you may recall, antioxidants generally become inactive after they have neutralized free radicals; they no longer have electrons to donate. By donating its own electrons to vitamin E, vitamin C restores vitamin E's antioxidant power, enabling it to continue its efforts to neutralize free radicals.

SUPPLEMENTS

Q: I'm considering boosting my intake of vitamin C with supplements. What's out there?

A: Quite a bit. Individual vitamin C supplements are available in a number of forms, brands and doses. Vitamin C is also available in combination with other nutrients— as part of a multivitamin or antioxidant supplement, for example.

Q: I'm not too familiar with multivitamin supplements. What types of vitamins do they contain and in what amounts?

A: Multivitamin and mineral supplements contain any number of vitamins and minerals in varying doses. Most multivitamin and mineral supplements contain some, but not all, of the nutrients for which RDAs have been set, in varying amounts. They may also contain varying amounts of nutrients for which no RDA has been established.

Q: What type of multivitamin and mineral supplement do the experts recommend?

A: While not all nutrition experts advocate nutritional supplements, many do believe that a multivitamin and mineral supplement can serve as "insurance" that you are getting enough of all the essential vitamins and minerals. These experts generally suggest that you buy a supplement that provides 100 percent of the RDA of the nutrients that have an RDA.

Q: Do any multivitamin and mineral supplements contain more than the RDA of certain nutrients?

A: Yes. Some do offer high amounts of antioxidants such as vitamins C and E and beta carotene. But it is easy enough, and sometimes cheaper, to simply purchase individual supplements of these vitamins.

Q: I'd like to know more about individual vitamin C supplements. In what forms are they available?

A: Vitamin C is available in two separate forms—as ascorbic acid and as mineral ascorbates, combinations of ascorbic acid and one or more minerals.

Q: Why would vitamin C be combined with minerals?

A: Because the minerals buffer vitamin C. Remember: Vitamin C is an acid. It can be hard on the stomach. Mineral ascorbates are gentler on the stomach, which makes them better for people who have difficulty taking straight ascorbic acid.

Q: How can you tell which form of vitamin C is in the supplement?

A: By reading the label. If ascorbic acid is listed in the ingredients, the supplement contains pure vitamin C. If the ingredients list calcium ascorbate, magnesium ascorbate or any other mineral in combination with the word "ascorbate," the supplement contains buffered vitamin C.

Q: How are all these vitamin C supplements sold? In pills?

A: Vitamin C supplements come in tablets, chewable tablets, effervescent tablets, extended-release tablets, extended-release capsules, powders, oral solutions and syrups. Vitamin C can also be given by injection.

Q: Which is best?

A: That's primarily a matter of personal preference. Size, taste and ability to swallow may make one form preferable over the others, but several forms do have a distinct disadvantage.

Q: What's that?

A: Because of their acidity, both the chewable tablets and the powder, which is dissolved in liquid then drunk, can cause the pH of the saliva to fall, damaging tooth enamel. In the case of the powder, this problem can be overcome if the liquid is sipped through a straw.

Q: I've heard people say that there's a difference between natural and synthetic vitamin supplements. Is there?

A: There is a difference, but in the case of vitamin C, it does not appear that either form has an advantage over the other. The difference is primarily in the way the supplements are made.

Natural vitamins are derived from foods, while synthetic vitamins are constructed from organic molecules found in an array of natural substances (in the case of vitamin C, these substances include starch, molasses and sago palm). In some cases, the distinction between natural and synthetic vitamin C is somewhat blurry. Vitamin C supplements containing rose hips (the seed pods of roses) are often labeled natural, but most supplements "with rose hips" actually contain very little natural vitamin C. Although rose hips do contain 1 percent vitamin C, because they are small, a vitamin C supplement made entirely of rose hips would be very large and very expensive. Consequently, supplement manufacturers combine the natural vitamin C with synthetic vitamin C.

> *Rose hips are a good source of vitamin C. A 1 ounce serving of these seed pods, which form after petals fall off of roses, can contain up to 300 milligrams of vitamin C. Pick hips as soon as they turn red; cut them open; remove and discard the seeds.*

Q: Does the source of the vitamin really matter?

A: It doesn't appear to. Studies have found that synthetic vitamin C and natural food sources of vitamin C are equally bioavailable.

Q: Are there any vitamin C supplements that include other compatible nutrients?

A: Yes. Vitamin C supplements are also sold with added **bioflavonoids**, nutrients found in plant-based foods that are thought to have antioxidant capabilities.

Q: Why?

A: The claim is that bioflavonoids, or **flavonoids**, as they're often called, enhance the absorption and use of vitamin C, but there is no evidence that this is the case. In fact, a study published in the July 1994 *Journal of the American Dietetic Association* compared three commercially available forms of synthetic vitamin C—ascorbic acid, ascorbic acid with bioflavonoids and an ascorbate sold under the brand name Ester-C—and found that the bioavailability was essentially the same in all of them.

"Our results have economic implications," the researchers wrote. "Tablets of Ester-C and ascorbic acid with bioflavonoids were 3.3 to 4.2 times more expensive than the ascorbic acid tablets."

Q: So is it bad to take these supplements?

A: Not necessarily. In fact, several studies suggest that bioflavonoids do have activity in the body; they may act as antioxidants and may possess antiviral and anti-inflammatory properties. But they apparently don't enhance the absorption and use of vitamin C as has been claimed.

Q: What about Ester-C? I thought I read somewhere that it was better than regular vitamin C.

A: Several earlier studies on Ester-C, the product of a patented process that combines ascorbic acid, calcium carbonate and distilled water, did indicate that it enters the bloodstream faster and remains in the body longer than plain ascorbic acid. But the *Journal of the American Dietetic Association* study found that blood levels of vitamin C were lower in the Ester-C group than in the ascorbic acid or ascorbic acid with bioflavonoids group at the time study participants' blood was tested. Blood levels of vitamin C in the Ester-C group also returned to their starting point faster.

What this means is that it is not clear whether Ester-C has any real advantage over plain vitamin C other than the fact that it is buffered and may be easier on the stomach.

Q: Let's say I decided to buy a regular vitamin C supplement. Should I go for the name brand, or is the store brand OK?

A: Many store brands are similar in formulation to expensive brand-name vitamins, but they cost much less. Check and compare labels to see what you are getting for your money. If a manufacturer claims its product is more readily absorbed or better balanced, you may want to contact the company and ask for research that backs up such marketing claims.

Q: Speaking about absorption, is there any way I can tell if the supplements I'm buying will dissolve properly and be absorbed?

A: Look for the letters "U.S.P." on the label. This means that the supplement meets manufacturing standards set by the U.S. Pharmacopoeia, an independent, nonprofit organization that sets standards for strength, quality, purity, packaging and labeling for medical products used in the United States.

To meet U.S.P. standards, water-soluble vitamins such as vitamin C should disintegrate in an environment that stimulates the digestive tract within 30 minutes if they're uncoated or 45 minutes if they're coated.

You can also help your body absorb the nutrients in a supplement by taking it at the end of a meal. The digestive juices stimulated by food help the supplement break down and be absorbed.

Q: **Is there any way I can make sure that the supplement I'm buying is fresh and at full potency?**

A: There's no way to be absolutely certain. Some supplement labels contain expiration dates beyond which you should not buy the product. Look for these dates. If no dates appear, look instead for a product that has good outer and inner seals.

Q: **How should I store my supplements?**

A: Keep your supplements in an opaque container rather than a clear one, and store the container in a dry, dark place away from sunlight and heat, making sure the lid is tightly sealed. Air, sunlight and dampness can affect their potency.

Q: **You said that taking supplements with food can help them be absorbed. Are there any other things I should know about taking vitamin C supplements?**

A: Yes. Because vitamin C is water soluble, it is not stored by the body. Consequently, many experts recommend that you spread your total vitamin C intake over the course of the day. This can help ensure a more constant blood level of vitamin C and, if you're taking large doses, help reduce the likelihood of adverse effects.

DIETARY SOURCES

Q: **What about the vitamin C found in foods? Is it any better than the vitamin C found in supplements?**

A: As we mentioned, studies have shown that both natural and synthetic vitamin C are equally absorbed and used by the body, but dietary vitamin C may still have an advantage—one that may not be directly related to the vitamin itself.

Q: **What is that?**

A: The vitamin C found in foods is rarely found alone. Other nutrients, too, are present in foods, notably other vitamins, minerals, bioflavonoids, fiber and other beneficial substances.

Q: **Is that why so many experts recommend that we get our vitamins from food?**

A: It's a major reason, yes. Foods (in this case, fruits and vegetables) provide a more complete package than do supplements—even multivitamin and mineral supplements. The combinations of nutrients foods provide—and possibly the way they work together—pack a big punch. Study after study shows the health benefits of diets high in fruit and vegetables.

The following herbs contain vitamin C:
- *burdock root*
- *goldenseal*
- *nettle*
- *chickweed*
- *rose hips*
- *eyebright*
- *yarrow*

Q: Is it possible to get adequate amounts of all the vitamins and minerals from food?

A: Some experts believe it's possible if you eat a balanced diet, but few Americans eat well enough to get the recommended amounts of nutrients each day from diet alone.

Q: What about vitamin C? Is it possible to get enough of that from the diet?

A: It depends on what you mean by enough. It's very easy to meet the 60-milligram RDA through food. One glass of orange or grapefruit juice or one-half cup of cooked broccoli will do the trick. And people who follow the government's recommendation to get at least five servings of fruits and vegetables per day will likely hit the 200-milligram mark recommended by researchers at the National Institutes of Health. But supplements are generally needed to achieve higher doses.

> *The following culinary herbs contain vitamin C:*
> * *cayenne*
> * *dandelion*
> * *fennel*
> * *garlic*
> * *green tea*
> * *horehound*
> * *parsley*
> * *peppermint*
> * *thyme*

Q: You mentioned orange juice. Is that any better than an orange?

A: Actually, the orange itself may be the better bet. A typical orange contains about 66 milligrams of vitamin C; a glass of orange juice may contain more or less, depending on how fresh it is and whether it has been fortified with vitamin C.

Q: What do you mean, depending on how fresh it is?

A: Freshly squeezed orange juice contains more vitamin C than orange juice that was squeezed some time in the past or prepared orange juice that has not been fortified.

Q: Why is that?

A: Because vitamin C is easily destroyed by air, light and heat. The amount of vitamin C in foods decreases rapidly during transport, processing, storage and preparation. Cutting, or even bruising, a fruit or vegetable can destroy some of the vitamin.

> *Snap beans cut into 1-inch pieces retain almost twice as much vitamin C as French-cut beans.*

Q: So I take it fresh fruits and vegetables are higher in vitamin C than processed ones?

A: Yes. Unless the processed fruits and vegetables have been fortified with vitamin C.

Q: What about cooking. Does that do anything to the vitamin C content of foods?

A: Yes. As we said, vitamin C is destroyed by both air and heat, so cooking vegetables reduces their vitamin C content. Boiling is particularly troublesome as the vitamin simply leaches into the cooking water.

Q: Are there any ways to ensure that I'm getting the most vitamin C out of my foods?

A: Yes. For maximum vitamin value, use fresh, unprocessed fruits and vegetables whenever possible; prepare fruits and vegetables as close as possible to the cooking time; serve foods as close as possible to the cooking time; and keep leftover food covered to avoid exposure to air.

Q: Is there anything else I need to know about vitamin C?

A: We've covered the basics. But as you know, new information on health and nutrition becomes available every day. Be alert to new findings on the roles vitamin C plays in the body, the vitamin's potential health benefits and new dosage recommendations to keep yourself up-to-date on this popular and beneficial nutrient.

GLOSSARY

Amino acids: Organic acids that make up proteins and are, thus, essential to life.

Angioplasty: A procedure for treating a narrowing or blockage of a blood vessel or heart valve. A catheter with a deflated balloon on its tip is passed into the narrowed artery segment, the balloon is inflated, and the narrow segment widened.

Antibodies: Substances made by the immune system to neutralize antigens.

Antigens: Substances foreign to the body that cause the immune system to form antibodies to neutralize them.

Antioxidants: Substances with the ability to interfere with oxygen-generated, or oxidative, reactions. These substances neutralize free radicals, unstable atomic or molecular fragments that can damage cells. Nutrients that act as antioxidants include vitamins C and E, beta carotene and selenium.

Ascorbate: See **Vitamin C.**

Ascorbic acid: See **Vitamin C.**

Atherosclerosis: A condition in which the inner layers of the artery walls become thick and irregular due to deposits of fat, cholesterol and other substances.

B lymphocytes: White blood cells that trigger the production of antibodies.

Bile acids: Acids produced during the breakdown of cholesterol; the forms in which excess cholesterol is eliminated from the body.

Bioavailability: The degree to which a nutrient or other substance becomes available for use in the body after ingestion or injection.

Bioflavonoids: Substances found in fruits that have been shown to have antioxidant properties.

Bipolar disorder: See **Manic depression**.

Bowel intolerance: The dosage of a vitamin at which gastrointestinal side effects occur.

Carotenoids: Any of a group of red, yellow or orange pigments that are found in foods such as carrots, sweet potatoes and leafy green vegetables. The body converts these substances to vitamin A.

Cataracts: Cloudings of the lens of the eye that obstruct vision.

Cell-mediated immunity: The type of immunity granted by T lymphocytes that helps the body resist infection.

Cholesterol: A white, waxy substance found naturally throughout the body, belonging to a class of compounds called sterols. Cholesterol is needed by the body to make hormones, vitamin D and bile acids and to build cells.

Collagen: A protein found in connective tissue, cartilage and bone. Collagen helps support and maintain the structure of tissue, including skin, muscles, gums, blood vessels and bones.

Coronary-artery disease: Atherosclerosis (blockage) of the coronary arteries, the spaghetti-size arteries that deliver blood to the heart.

Diabetes: A disease resulting from the body's inability to produce or use insulin, resulting in high blood sugar levels.

Dietary Reference Intakes (DRIs): Dietary recommendations made by the National Academy of Sciences. These recommendations, which include four categories of reference intakes, are intended to replace the Recommended Dietary Allowances. They include Recommended Dietary Allowances, Adequate Intakes, Estimated Average Requirements and Tolerable Upper Intake Levels.

DRIs: See **Dietary Reference Intakes (DRIs).**

Endothelium: A layer of cells that lines and protects the inner surfaces of blood vessels.

Epidemiologic studies: Studies to determine the distribution and causes of various health problems. These studies involve surveillance, observation, hypothesis-testing and experimentation.

Epinephrine: A hormone that is secreted during stress of any kind; also known as adrenaline.

Fibrinogen: A protein in blood plasma that aids in the clotting process.

Flavonoids: See **Bioflavonoids.**

Free radicals: Molecular fragments that attempt to steal electrons from other molecules. Free radicals have been linked to a number of chronic diseases, including heart disease and cancer.

Gout: A form of arthritis caused by deposits of uric acid crystals in joints.

HDL: See **High-density lipoprotein (HDL).**

High-density lipoprotein (HDL): The so-called good cholesterol that helps to escort cholesterol from the body. High levels are linked with reduced risk for heart disease.

Histamine: A biochemical released by the immune system that widens blood vessels, lowers blood pressure, releases gastric juices, contracts smooth muscles and irritates nerve endings.

Humoral immunity: The form of immunity provided by the development and presence of antibodies.

Hypertension: A chronic increase in blood pressure above its normal range; generally, systolic readings greater than 140 mm Hg and/or diastolic readings greater than 90 mm Hg over a period of time.

Immune response: The manner in which the immune system protects the body from disease. There are two types of immune response: humoral and cell-mediated.

Immune system: The complex system that protects the body from disease organisms and other foreign bodies; includes the humoral immune response and the cell-mediated immune response.

Insulin: A hormone produced in the pancreas that enables the body to use sugar for energy.

Interferon: Any of a class of small proteins that exert antiviral activity on cells. They also regulate many cell properties and functions.

LDL: See **Low-density lipoprotein (LDL)**.

Leukocytes: White blood cells.

Lipid peroxidation: Oxidation of fats in the body; an early step in the development of atherosclerosis.

Low-density lipoprotein (LDL): The so-called bad cholesterol. High levels of LDL cholesterol have been linked with increased risk for heart disease.

Lymphokines: Chemicals produced and released by T lymphocytes that attract phagocytes to the site of an infection or inflammation.

Macula: Central area of the retina responsible for sharp, fine vision.

Macular degeneration: Damage or breakdown of the macula; a leading cause of blindness.

Manic depression: A disorder in which bouts of major depression alternate with mania, a condition characterized by energetic, risk-taking, impulsive and often self-destructive behavior; also known as bipolar disorder.

Mediators: Chemicals that mediate, or act on, various components of the immune system; these chemicals provoke inflammation and cause the symptoms of allergic reactions.

Megadoses: Nutrient doses that are 10 times the RDA.

Mineral: A nonorganic compound, one that doesn't contain carbon and does not originate from living organisms.

Nephropathy: Kidney disease or damage leading to kidney failure; a complication of diabetes.

Nitrosamines: Potentially carcinogenic substances formed in the digestive tract from nitrates and nitrites.

Norepinephrine: A neurotransmitter found in the brain, released during stress. Low levels of norepinephrine have been linked to depression; also known as noradrenaline.

Nutrient: A substance used by the body that must be supplied from foods consumed. The six classes of nutrients are water, proteins, carbohydrates, fats, minerals and vitamins.

Osteoarthritis: Degenerative arthritis, often caused by joint injuries or old age. The most common type of arthritis.

Oxalate: A salt of oxalic acid found in the urine; its presence in the urine increases with increased vitamin C intake, possibly raising the risk of kidney stones.

Oxalic acid: An acid found in plants and vegetables; its salts are found in urine and may contribute to kidney stones.

Oxidation: A chemical process in which a molecule combines with oxygen and loses electrons. Antioxidant nutrients such as vitamins C and E help control oxidation.

Phagocytes: Immune cells that engulf and ingest foreign invaders.

Placebo: An inactive substance.

Plaque: A deposit of fatty (and other) substances in the inner lining of an artery wall characteristic of atherosclerosis.

Plasma: The fluid portion of blood.

Platelets: Small, disk-shaped structures involved in blood coagulation.

Polyps: Masses of tissue that bulge or project outward or upward from the normal surface level.

Pro-oxidant: Promoting oxidation.

Pulmonary function tests: Tests that determine how well the lungs are performing and estimate the severity of airway obstruction.

RDA: See **Recommended Dietary Allowance (RDA)**.

Recommended Dietary Allowance (RDA): The levels of intake of essential nutrients that, on the basis of scientific knowledge, are judged by the National Academy of Sciences' Food and Nutrition Board to be adequate to meet the known nutrient needs of practically all healthy persons.

Retinopathy: A disease of the blood vessels of the retina, the light-sensing surface on the rear wall of the eye; a complication of diabetes.

Schizophrenia: A psychotic disorder characterized by loss of contact with the environment and by disordered feelings and thoughts.

Scurvy: A vitamin C-deficiency disease characterized by bleeding gums, pink or red hemorrhagic spots under the skin, rough skin, joint pain, fatigue, tissue degeneration and increased incidence of infection.

Serotonin: A neurotransmitter that controls states of consciousness, mood, sleep and sensitivity to pain.

Sorbitol: A sugar alcohol produced in the body during the conversion of glucose.

Stroke: A sudden loss of function of part of the brain due to an interference in blood supply.

Supplements: Vitamins, minerals and other nutrients taken either alone or in combination to "supplement" the amount received through the diet.

T lymphocytes: White blood cells responsible for cell-mediated immunity.

Thymus: A gland that is part of the immune system; where T lymphocytes mature.

Triglycerides: Fatty compounds found in the blood that contain three chains of fat and one glycerol (alcohol) module.

Tryptophan: An amino acid; vitamin C helps convert tryptophan into serotonin.

Tyrosine: An amino acid that contributes to the formation of epinephrine and norepinephrine.

Urate: A salt of uric acid.

Uric acid: A crystalline substance found in urine.

Vasodilators: Drugs that cause the muscle in the walls of blood vessels to relax, allowing the artery to dilate, or widen.

Vitamin C: A water-soluble vitamin with strong antioxidant properties; also known as ascorbate or ascorbic acid.

Vitamins: Organic components of food found to be essential in small quantities for normal human metabolism, growth and physical well-being.

Water soluble: Able to be dissolved in water. The water-soluble vitamins—the B vitamins and vitamin C—are not stored in the body but are quickly excreted; they must be replenished regularly.

INDEX